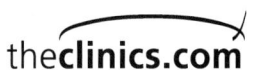

ORTHOPEDIC CLINICS OF NORTH AMERICA

Patellofemoral Arthritis

GUEST EDITOR
Wayne B. Leadbetter, MD

July 2008 • Volume 39 • Number 3

SAUNDERS

An Imprint of Elsevier, Inc.
PHILADELPHIA LONDON TORONTO MONTREAL SYDNEY TOKYO

W.B. SAUNDERS COMPANY
A Division of Elsevier Inc.

Elsevier Inc., 1600 John F. Kennedy Blvd., Suite 1800, Philadelphia, PA 19103-2899.

http://www.orthopedic.theclinics.com

ORTHOPEDIC CLINICS OF NORTH AMERICA
July 2008
Editor: Debora Dellapena

Volume 39, Number 3
ISSN 0030-5898
ISBN-10: 1-4160-6330-7
ISBN-13: 978-1-4160-6330-8

© 2008 Elsevier ■ All rights reserved.

This journal and the individual contributions contained in it are protected under copyright by Elsevier, and the following terms and conditions apply to their use:

Photocopying
Single photocopies of single articles may be made for personal use as allowed by national copyright laws. Permission of the Publisher and payment of a fee is required for all other photocopying, including multiple or systematic copying, copying for advertising or promotional purposes, resale, and all forms of document delivery. Special rates are available for educational institutions that wish to make photocopies for non-profit educational classroom use. For information on how to seek permission visit www.elsevier.com/permissions or call: (+44) 1865 843830 (UK)/(+1) 215 239 3804 (USA).

Derivative Works
Subscribers may reproduce tables of contents or prepare lists of articles including abstracts for internal circulation within their institutions. Permission of the Publisher is required for resale or distribution outside the institution. Permission of the Publisher is required for all other derivative works, including compilations and translations (please consult www.elsevier.com/permissions).

Electronic Storage or Usage
Permission of the Publisher is required to store or use electronically any material contained in this journal, including any article or part of an article (please consult www.elsevier.com/permissions). Except as outlined above, no part of this publication may be reproduced, stored in a retrieval system or transmitted in any form or by any means, electronic, mechanical, photocopying, recording or otherwise, without prior written permission of the Publisher.

Notice
No responsibility is assumed by the Publisher for any injury and/or damage to persons or property as a matter of products liability, negligence or otherwise, or from any use or operation of any methods, products, instructions or ideas contained in the material herein. Because of rapid advances in the medical sciences, in particular, independent verification of diagnoses and drug dosages should be made. Although all advertising material is expected to conform to ethical (medical) standards, inclusion in this publication does not constitute a guarantee or endorsement of the quality or value of such product or of the claims made of it by its manufacturer.

Orthopedic Clinics of North America (ISSN 0030-5898) is published quarterly (For Post Office use only: Volume 39 issue 3 of 4) by Elsevier Inc., 360 Park Avenue South, New York, NY 10010-1710. Months of publication are January, April, July, and October. Business and Editorial Offices: 1600 John F. Kennedy Blvd., Suite 1800, Philadelphia, PA 19103-2899. Customer Service Office: 6277 Sea Harbor Drive, Orlando, FL 33887-4800. Periodicals postage paid at New York, NY and additional mailing offices. Subscription prices are $226.00 per year for (US individuals), $389.00 per year for (US institutions), $267.00 per year (Canadian individuals), $456.00 per year (Canadian institutions), $309.00 per year (international individuals), $456.00 per year (international institutions), $113.00 per year (US students), $154.00 per year (Canadian and international students). Foreign air speed delivery is included in all *Clinics* subscription prices. All prices are subject to change without notice. **POSTMASTER:** Send address changes to *Orthopedic Clinics of North America*, Elsevier Periodicals Customer Service, 6277 Sea Harbor Drive, Orlando, FL 32887-4800. **Customer Service: 1-800-654-2452 (US). From outside the United States, call 1-407-563-6020. Fax: 1-407-363-9661. E-mail: JournalsCustomerService-usa@elsevier.com.**

Reprints. For copies of 100 or more of articles in this publication, please contact the Commercial Reprints Department, Elsevier Inc., 360 Park Avenue South, New York, NY 10010-1710. Tel.: 212-633-3812; Fax: 212-462-1935; E-mail: reprints@elsevier.com.

Orthopedic Clinics of North America is covered in MEDLINE/PubMed (*Index Medicus*), Cinahl, Excerpta Medica, and Cumulative Index to Nursing and Allied Health Literature.

Printed in the United States of America.

Right cover image: Leadbetter WB, Seyler TM, Ragland PS, et al. Indications, contraindications, and pitfalls of patellofemoral arthroplasty. J Bone Joint Surg Am 2006;88(Suppl 4):133.

PATELLOFEMORAL ARTHRITIS

GUEST EDITOR

WAYNE B. LEADBETTER, MD, Center for Joint Preservation and Replacement, Rubin Institute for Advanced Orthopedics, Sinai Hospital of Baltimore, Baltimore, Maryland

CONTRIBUTORS

JACK ANDRISH, MD, Department of Orthopaedic Surgery, Cleveland Clinic Foundation, Cleveland Clinic, Cleveland, Ohio

ERIN BAKER, MPT, PT, Team Leader, Outpatient Physical Therapy, Rubin Institute for Advanced Orthopedics, Sinai Hospital, Sinai Hospital, Baltimore, Maryland

ANIL BHAVE, PT, Division Head of Rehabilitation; Director of Wasserman Gait Laboratory, Rubin Institute for Advanced Orthopedics, Sinai Hospital; Assistant Clinical Professor, Department of Physical Therapy, University of Maryland, Baltimore, Maryland

PETER M. BONUTTI, MD, Bonutti Clinic, Effingham, Illinois

PHILIP A. DAVIDSON, MD, Tampa Bay Orthopaedic Specialists; Department of Orthopaedic Surgery, University of South Florida, Pinellas Park, Florida

DAVID DEJOUR, MD, Corolyon Sauvegarde, Lyon, France

RONALD E. DELANOIS, MD, Center for Joint Preservation and Reconstruction, Rubin Institute for Advanced Orthopedics, Sinai Hospital of Baltimore, Baltimore, Maryland

JACK FARR, II, MD, OrthoIndy Knee Care Institute; Voluntary Associate Clinical Professor of Orthopaedic Surgery, Indiana University School of Medicine, Indianapolis, Indiana

JASON GOULD, MD, Resident, Department of Orthopedic Surgery, The Mount Sinai Medical Center, New York, New York

RONALD P. GRELSAMER, MD, Associate Professor of Orthopedic Surgery; Chief, Patellofemoral Reconstruction, The Mount Sinai Medical Center, New York, New York

WAYNE B. LEADBETTER, MD, Center for Joint Preservation and Replacement, Rubin Institute for Advanced Orthopedics, Sinai Hospital of Baltimore, Baltimore, Maryland

JESS H. LONNER, MD, Director, Knee Replacement Surgery, Booth Bartolozzi Balderston Orthopaedics, Pennsylvania Hospital, Philadelphia, Pennsylvania

DAVID R. MARKER, BS, Center for Joint Preservation and Reconstruction, Rubin Institute for Advanced Orthopedics, Sinai Hospital of Baltimore, Baltimore, Maryland

MIKE S. McGRATH, MD, Center for Joint Preservation and Reconstruction, Rubin Institute for Advanced Orthopedics, Sinai Hospital of Baltimore, Baltimore, Maryland

MICHAEL A. MONT, MD, Center for Joint Preservation and Reconstruction, Rubin Institute for Advanced Orthopedics, Sinai Hospital of Baltimore, Baltimore, Maryland

DENNIS RIVENBURGH, MS, ATC, PA-C, Tampa Bay Orthopaedic Specialists, Pinellas Park, Florida

VINEET K. SARIN, PhD, Kinamed Incorporated, Camarillo, California

THORSTEN M. SEYLER, MD, Center for Joint Preservation and Reconstruction, Rubin Institute for Advanced Orthopedics, Sinai Hospital of Baltimore, Baltimore, Maryland

DOMENICK J. SISTO, MD, Los Angeles Orthopaedic Institute, Sherman Oaks, California

ROBERT A. TEITGE, MD, Professor, Department of Orthopaedic Surgery, Wayne State University, School of Medicine, Detroit, Michigan

SLIF D. ULRICH, MD, Center for Joint Preservation and Reconstruction, Rubin Institute for Advanced Orthopedics, Sinai Hospital of Baltimore, Baltimore, Maryland

CONTENTS

Preface ix
Wayne B. Leadbetter

The Pathophysiology of Patellofemoral Arthritis 269
Ronald P. Grelsamer, David Dejour, and Jason Gould

> Faced with a patient suffering from patellofemoral arthritis, the surgeon must determine the pathophysiology of the condition, because different causes demand different treatments. Possible causes include malalignment, patellofemoral dysplasia, patellofemoral instability, patellofemoral trauma, obesity, osteoarthritis, inflammatory arthritis, and a genetic predisposition. Arthritis secondary to malalignment, dysplasia, instability, or trauma is less likely than arthritis secondary to the other causes to progress to femorotibial arthritis.

Prescribing Quality Patellofemoral Rehabilitation Before Advocating Operative Care 275
Anil Bhave and Erin Baker

> In this article we discuss causes of patellofemoral dysfunction, the treatment algorithm of nonsurgical therapy modalities, and what constitutes a quality rehabilitation protocol for a patient with patellofemoral dysfunction.

Patellofemoral Syndrome a Paradigm for Current Surgical Strategies 287
Robert A. Teitge

> The literature regarding suggested treatments for patellofemoral problems is often conflicting and confusing. In this discussion I present the approach I take in evaluating and considering surgery for patients with any of a wide variety of anterior knee pain problems. It has been useful to concentrate on the biomechanics—the mechanical consequence to each tissue affected by any surgical change. In the proposed paradigm, it is assumed that pain is the result of an abnormal load—related either to tension or compression—being applied to each tissue in question. The challenge is to understand how and why that abnormal load was generated. It is essential to make an independent assessment of the condition of the lower limb skeleton, the patellofemoral ligaments, and the trochlear and patellar articular cartilage in each patient. While only a long book can address this subject in detail, this discussion provides a guide for formulating an analysis of the key issues when planning the operative treatment of patellofemoral pain and dysfunction.

The Management of Recurrent Patellar Dislocation 313
Jack Andrish

Acute and chronic trauma, chronic abnormal joint loading conditions, and hemarthroses have been implicated in the development of degenerative joint disease. Patellar instability with acute and recurrent patellar dislocation provides all of these ingredients. This article describes an approach to the treatment of recurrent patellar instability that considers the unique features and expectations of the patient rather than using a generic algorithm.

Autologous Chondrocyte Implantation and Anteromedialization in the Treatment of Patellofemoral Chondrosis 329
Jack Farr, II

Patellofemoral articular cartilage lesions are challenging to treat. While treatment with tibial tuberosity anteromedialization (AMZ) is effective for isolated distal lateral patellar lesions, other patellar or trochlear lesions have suboptimal outcomes with AMZ. Historically, when autologous cultured chondroctye implantation (ACI) was used at the patellofemoral compartment without optimizing the contact areas, the results were poor. In recent years, the combination of AMZ and ACI has yielded overall outcomes superior to either technique used in isolation for large patellar and trochlear chondral lesions.

Focal Anatomic Patellofemoral Inlay Resurfacing: Theoretic Basis, Surgical Technique, and Case Reports 337
Philip A. Davidson and Dennis Rivenburgh

Prosthetic patellofemoral inlay resurfacing is a novel treatment concept for degenerative and focal arthrosis of the patellofemoral joint. The theoretic basis of this type of arthroplasty entails recreating ambient anatomy based upon intraoperative topographic mapping. The implant is intrinsically stable by virtue of the inset position relative to the surrounding joint surface. Articular resurfacing, rather than traditional replacement arthroplasty, represents an extension of the concepts of biologic joint restoration. Early results have shown great efficacy. This surgery may be appropriate for a wide variety of indications, including younger patients and those with focal patellofemoral disease concurrent with morphologic or alignment abnormalities.

Patellofemoral Arthroplasty: The Impact of Design on Outcomes 347
Jess H. Lonner

The results of patellofemoral arthroplasty have been improved over the three decades that the procedure has been used for the treatment of patellofemoral arthritis. Specifically, there has been a reduction in the incidence of patellofemoral-related problems, such as patellar maltracking and catching, after patellofemoral arthroplasty. While these problems were often attributed to errors in surgical technique or component malposition, it is likely that many were related to flawed trochlear component designs. Contemporary patellofemoral arthroplasties have a reduced incidence of the problems related to patellar maltracking that typically plagued earlier generation designs. Further study will likely prove contemporary patellofemoral arthroplasty to be an effective treatment for the management of isolated patellofemoral arthritis, with predictable outcomes and a low incidence of complications.

Patellofemoral Arthroplasty with a Customized Trochlear Prosthesis 355
Domenick J. Sisto and Vineet K. Sarin

Successful patellofemoral arthroplasty depends on appropriate patient selection, proper prosthesis design, and correct surgical technique. Clinical results using off-the-shelf patellofemoral prostheses have reported mixed results primarily because of an inability to address these important characteristics adequately. This article reviews the design rationale, excellent clinical history, and straightforward surgical technique of a unique approach to patellofemoral arthroplasty that incorporates a customized trochlear prosthesis designed to fit the individual patient's patellofemoral groove. Clinical results using this customized approach demonstrate that it is a safe and effective treatment option for patients who have isolated patellofemoral arthritis.

Patellofemoral Arthroplasty in the Treatment of Patellofemoral Arthritis: Rationale and Outcomes in Younger Patients 363
Wayne B. Leadbetter

Patellofemoral degenerative disease encompasses a spectrum of articular wear from severe chondrosis to advanced arthrosis. The rationale and timing for many operative approaches currently advocated for the relief of symptomatic patellofemoral degeneration can be the subject of intense surgical debate in any one patient. Unfortunately, the limited efficacy of many commonly advocated operative procedures has left a legacy of patellofemoral disability in many younger individuals. While total knee arthroplasty has an established role in the treatment of advanced patellofemoral arthritis in the older patient (age >60 years), the performance of what some have called "a knee joint amputation" in younger patients (age <45 years) remains controversial and less acceptable to patients. The Avon patellofemoral prosthesis is a second-generation knee joint-conserving device that has consistently achieved good to excellent results in both the primary treatment and salvage of patellofemoral degenerative disease in younger patients. In addition, patellofemoral arthroplasty has demonstrated success as a unique functional, tibial-femoral joint-conserving solution in a variety of other patellofemoral extensor mechanism problems.

Results of Total Knee Replacement for Isolated Patellofemoral Arthritis: When Not to Perform a Patellofemoral Arthroplasty 381
Ronald E. Delanois, Mike S. McGrath, Slif D. Ulrich, David R. Marker, Thorsten M. Seyler, Peter M. Bonutti, and Michael A. Mont

Many procedures have been used to treat advanced isolated patellofemoral arthritis, with varying results. Patellofemoral arthroplasty (PFA) is a bone-conserving procedure that has shown short-term success but has relatively high revision rates. Total knee arthroplasty (TKA) has been recommended for treatment of this disease in patients who are older than 60 years of age. Recent literature indicates that PFA is most successful in patients who have isolated patellofemoral arthritis secondary to trochlear dysplasia or patellar fracture and in patients who are younger than 60 years; TKA is recommended for older patients who have primary or idiopathic isolated patellofemoral arthritis.

Index 389

FORTHCOMING ISSUES

October 2008
Shoulder Trauma
George S. Athwal, MD, FRCSC,
Guest Editor

January 2009
Spine Oncology
Rakesh Donthineni, MD, MBA
Onder Ofluoglu, MD, *Guest Editors*

April 2009
Bone Circulation Disorders
Michael A. Mont, MD, *Guest Editor*

RECENT ISSUES

April 2008
Elbow Trauma
Scott P. Steinmann, MD, *Guest Editor*

January 2008
Orthopedic Ancillary Services: A Guide to Practice Management
Jack M. Bert, MD, *Guest Editor*

October 2007
Scoliosis
Anthony A. Stans, MD, *Guest Editor*

The Clinics are now available online!

Access your subscription at:
http://www.theclinics.com

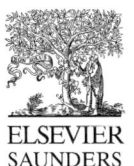

Preface

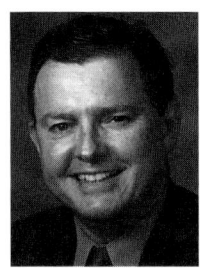

Wayne B. Leadbetter, MD
Guest Editor

"There are no heroes in patellofemoral surgery."
—Blazina, 1979

The operative treatment of the painful degenerative patellofemoral joint is challenging and controversial. This remains true despite long recognition that the refractory advanced stages of isolated patellofemoral chondrosis and arthrosis can and frequently do create prominent patient disability and limb dysfunction. In the past, too often the legacy of patellofemoral surgery has been one of ill-timed operations applied with inadequate rationale, resulting in iatrogenic outcomes. This had often left surgeons with the jaded view that "no patellofemoral complaints get better." The worn patellofemoral joint was relegated to the fate of benign neglect, patellectomy, or eventual total joint replacement.

Fortunately, times are changing. The renewed priority shown by orthopedic surgeons, researchers, rehabilitation specialists, biomechanists, and biotechnology innovators on conserving the patellofemoral joint, the so-called "forgotten joint," has grown exponentially in the current literature. The multiple factors that contribute to the onset of patellofemoral degeneration and arthritis have been better defined, including the importance of patellofemoral dysplasia and instability, extensor mechanism malalignment, and overall limb malalignment. These insights, along with recent advances in articular cartilage restoration techniques and isolated prosthetic resurfacing, offer more options for individualizing patellofemoral operative care. While Balzina's wise council should be cause to stop and be sure that our reach does not exceed our grasp, today's orthopedic surgeon is better equipped to cope with patellofemoral disorders.

The contributors to this issue have been engaged leaders in trying to prevent misadventures in patellofemoral arthritic surgery for both surgeon and patient while at the same time encouraging advances in operative approach. It is our intention to provide a balanced pragmatic understanding of how to better advise and surgically treat the patient with symptomatic, disabling, patellofemoral disease who has truly failed all reasonable alternatives.

Wayne B. Leadbetter, MD
Center for Joint Preservation and Replacement
Rubin Institute for Advanced Orthopedics
Sinai Hospital of Baltimore
2401 West Belvedere Avenue
Baltimore, MD 21215

E-mail address: wleadbet@lifebridgehealth.org

The Pathophysiology of Patellofemoral Arthritis

Ronald P. Grelsamer, MD[a,*], David Dejour, MD[b], Jason Gould, MD[c]

[a]Patellofemoral Reconstruction, The Mount Sinai Medical Center, Box 1188, 5 East 98th Street, New York, NY 10029, USA
[b]Corolyon Sauvegarde, 8 Avenue Ben Gourion, 69009 Lyon, France
[c]Department of Orthopedic Surgery, The Mount Sinai Medical Center, 5 East 98th Street, New York, NY 10029, USA

Faced with a patient suffering from patellofemoral arthritis, the surgeon must determine the pathophysiology of the condition, because different causes of patellofemoral arthritis demand different treatments. Specifically, before elaborating a treatment plan, the surgeon, to best of his or her ability, must determine whether the patellofemoral arthritis truly is isolated to the patellofemoral compartment, and, if so, if it is likely to remain isolated for the foreseeable future. For the purposes of this article, the term "arthritis" refers to a full-thickness loss of articular cartilage.

The articular cartilage of the patella is similar to all other articular cartilage in that it consists of a fluid phase and a solid phase that is made up mostly of collagen and glycosaminoglycans. The solid phase is somewhat permeable. When a load is applied to the articular surface, the fluid gradually redistributes itself within the solid matrix [1,2]. The pressure within the fluid is largely responsible for the cushioning effect of the articular cartilage and the low friction coefficient exhibited by articular surfaces. Any disruption of the articular surface (eg, by cracks, fissures, crevices, and the like) leads to a loss of pressure within the fluid phase. High stresses then are borne by the collagen fibers, which become more prone to breakdown [3]. The articular cartilage of the patella is much, thicker, softer, and more permeable than any other human articular cartilage, including that of the trochlea.

* Corresponding author.
 E-mail address: ronald.grelsamer@mountsinai.org (R.P. Grelsamer).

Certain causes of arthritis are associated with isolated patellofemoral arthritis; others are more likely to reflect a generalized knee condition.

Causes of patellofemoral arthritis include malalignment (abnormal tilt, abnormal Q angle, abnormal torsion), dysplasia (trochlear and patellar), instability, trauma, inflammatory arthritis, obesity, and osteoarthritis.

Malalignment

"Malalignment" is a general term encompassing conditions that lead to poor positioning and poor tracking of the patella. An improper fit of the mating surfaces leads to abnormal distributions of pressure, which in turn can lead to arthritis. Merchant and Mercer [4] in California and Ficat and colleagues [5] in France were the first to postulate that a tilted patella (lateral side down) associated with a tight lateral retinaculum would lead to excessive pressures at the lateral aspect of the patellofemoral compartment. Putz and colleagues [6] and Eckstein and colleagues [7] demonstrated CT scan evidence of hyper-pressure on the subchondral bone of the lateral patella in patients who had patellar tilt.

No prospective study has been undertaken to verify that patients who have malalignment have a greater predisposition to arthritis, but patients who have patellofemoral arthritis often demonstrate malalignment. Iwano and colleagues [8] reviewed 108 knees in 61 women and 5 men who had patellofemoral arthritis (with or without concomitant femorotibial arthritis). Twenty-eight percent of patients who had isolated patellofemoral arthritis (9/32) gave a history of patellar instability. In 59 of the 64 knees with isolated patellofemoral arthritis (92%), the arthritis was located at the lateral half of the patella.

A greatly increased (or decreased) Q angle could be expected to lead to increased pressures between the patella and the lateral (or medial) wall of the trochlea. Indeed, Goutallier and colleagues [9] have found increased pain in patients whose normally positioned tibial tuberosity is transposed medially. They also have introduced the concept of the Q angle as it relates to the trochlea. A patient who has a steep trochlea is more susceptible to increased patellar-trochlear pressures if the Q angle is significantly high or low. In their study the patients who experienced the greatest pain following tibial tuberosity transfers were those who had steep trochleas (< 140°) and low Q angles.

Abnormal distal femoral torsion—usually internal—brings excessive pressure to bear on the lateral aspect of the patellofemoral compartment and functionally is equivalent to patellar tilt.

Patients whose isolated patellofemoral arthritis is secondary to malalignment are good candidates for tibial tuberosity transfers and patellofemoral replacements, because the arthritis is not likely to progress to the other compartments. (Progression of arthritis to the femorotibial compartments is the main cause of failure in patellofemoral replacement surgery.)

Patellofemoral dysplasia

The patellofemoral articulation is unique in its great morphologic variability from person to person. Grelsamer and Meadows [10] studied the patella in the sagittal plane, and Henri Dejour and colleagues [11] and David Dejour and Le-Coultre [12] have studied the various forms of trochlear dysplasia.

The patellofemoral articulation is well suited to its function and usually does not break down, even though it is incongruent in the sagittal plane, with only a minority of the patella in contact with the trochlea at any given time [13]. On close inspection one notes that the articular cartilage of the patella features multiple facets in patterns that are unique to each patient [14]. The trochlea generally is U-shaped, the U beginning at the proximal portion of the trochlea and becoming progressively deeper. When imaged with the knee flexed 30° to 40°, the trochlea has an angle of approximately 140°.

The normal functioning of the patellofemoral joint depends on the smooth interplay of these complex geometries. When a variation occurs at the patella that is well matched by the trochlea, the forces remain well distributed, and the stresses remain within a tolerable range. Thus a trochlea that is slightly steeper or more shallow than usual can be tolerated, as long as the patella matches this variation.

Some trochlear variations, however, are so significant that even a matching patella may not provide adequate compensation. These variations include unusually steep or shallow trochleas and trochleas featuring an area of convexity proximally.

Patellofemoral dysplasia is highly correlated with patellofemoral arthritis, and there even is a specific correlation between arthritis and the various forms of dysplasia [15]. The diagnosis of trochlear dysplasia is made on a true lateral radiograph, on which the posterior aspects of the two femoral condyles appear superimposed [16]. The basic feature of dysplasia is the crossing sign, which is a convergence of the trochlea and of the lateral femoral condyle; on a normal trochlea, the two lines remain distinct to the origin of the trochlea [17]. The more distal the crossing, the more severe is the dysplasia.

Moreover, in more severe forms of dysplasia the trochlea is elevated anteriorly relative to the anterior cortex of the femur. This elevation is judged easily by virtually prolonging the anterior cortex distally on the lateral radiograph and by measuring the position of the trochlea relative to this projection.

In some patients, the proximal trochlea also features a bony spur that projects anteriorly, the supratrochlear spur.

A linear cortical projection of the anterior cortex into the mass of the condyles, the double contour sign, indicates advanced dysplasia of the medial wall of the trochlea (Figs. 1 and 2) [1,2,12].

Trochlear dysplasia can be classified into four categories based on these characteristics (Fig. 3) [12,18].

Part of the dysplastic process can include patella alta, and one should remember to check the various parameters of patellar height (Fig. 4) [19]. In a study of 367 patients who had isolated patellofemoral arthritis, Dejour and Allain [15] noted that patellofemoral dysplasia was the most common predisposing factor. Indeed, 78% of patients had a positive crossing sign on the lateral radiograph.

Trochlear dysplasia was noted in 96% of patients who had a history of one or more documented dislocations but was present in only 3% of a control population [11,20].

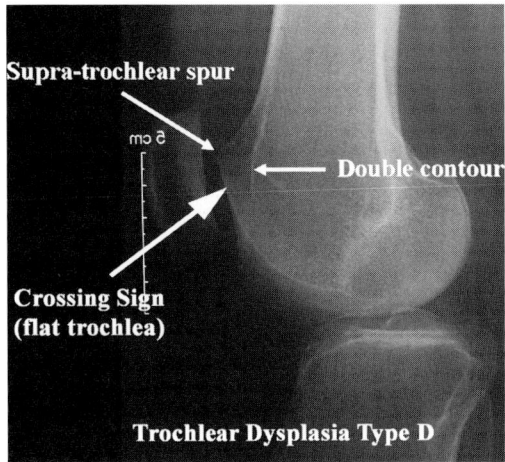

Fig. 1. This lateral radiograph exemplifies many possible elements of trochlear dysplasia: the crossing sign (flat trochlea), the supratrochlear spur, the anterior position of the proximal trochlea, and the abnormal projection of the medial trochlear wall.

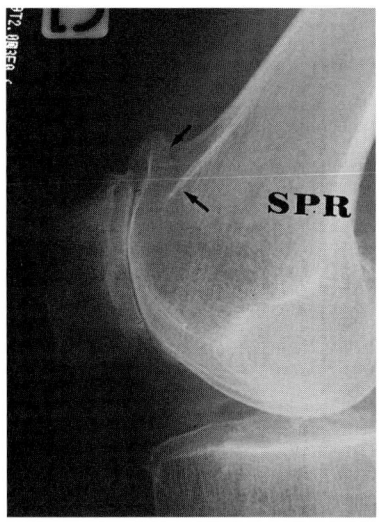

Fig. 2. Isolated patellofemoral arthritis in a patient who has type D dysplasia.

Dysplasia represents the link between patellar instability and the risk of patellofemoral arthritis. Patients who have category B, C, and D dysplasia (patients in whom the proximal trochlea is anterior to the distal femoral cortex and/or patients who have a spur at the proximal trochlea) are at greatest risk [12].

The degree of arthritis (according to the classification of Iwano and colleagues [8]) correlates with the degree of dysplasia: the greater the dysplasia and the more anterior the trochlea lies relative to the distal femur, the greater is the arthritis ($P = .0046$) (Table 1) [15].

The prominence of the proximal trochlea presumably has a reverse Maquet effect by increasing

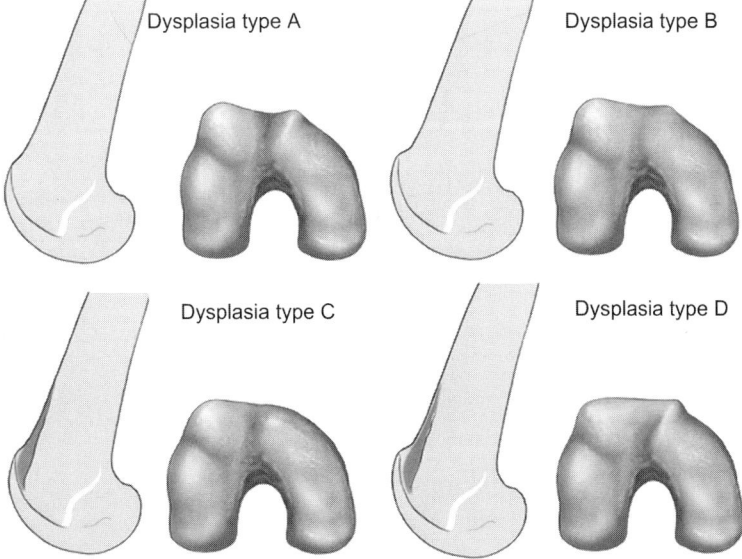

Fig. 3. Dejour's classification of trochlear dysplasia classification. Type A: crossing sign (flat or convex trochlea). Type B: crossing sign and supratrochlear spur. Type C: crossing sign and double contour. Type D: crossing sign, supratrochlear spur, double contour, and sharp step-off of the trochlea.

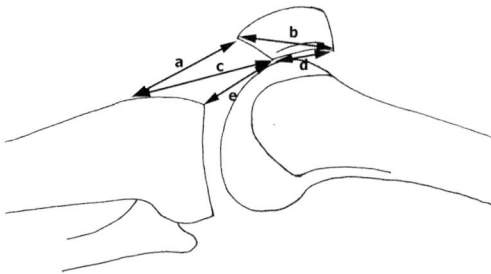

Fig. 4. Measurements of patellar height: Insall-Salvati (a/b), Modified Insall-Salvati (c/d), Blackburne and Peel (approximate) and Caton-Deschamps (e/d).

the patellofemoral pressures, and the deformation of the trochlear anatomy further distorts patellofemoral relationships (eg, tilt and pressure distributions).

The "kissing" lesions seen in the central portion of the patella and over the lateral aspect of the trochlea in patients who have a history of patellar dislocation probably represent precursors to arthritis.

Isolated patellofemoral arthritis is seen at slightly earlier ages in patients who have trochlear dysplasia than in patients who have patellofemoral arthritis of other causes (54 years versus 56 years), and high-grade dysplasia is more prevalent in the instability/arthritis category (66%) than in the asymptomatic category (38%) [15].

Patella alta as an isolated factor was not found to predispose to arthritis.

Instability (symptomatic medial-lateral displacement, including dislocation)

Although the patellofemoral compartment is not congruent when viewed in the sagittal plane, it is congruent in the axial plane. Because the articulation is roughly U-shaped, any medial-lateral displacement of the patella results in abnormal shear stresses at the articular surface.

The association between subluxation of the patella (partial loss of congruence in the axial plane) and arthritis has not been studied formally, but arthritis following frank patellar dislocation has been the subject of a few studies, many of which originate in Finland [21–23]. Patients suffering from a single dislocation have a higher rate of arthritis than patients who have multiple dislocations. Patients who have recurrent dislocations are more likely to exhibit an anatomy that facilitates these dislocations. Less force is required to dislocate the patella in these patients than in patients who suffer only one dislocation. The situation is somewhat analogous to shoulder instability.

A study by Maenpaa and Lehto [22] demonstrated a higher rate of arthritis in patients who had undergone surgical treatment for instability than in patients treated nonoperatively. The spectrum of surgical procedures used in these patients, however, includes procedures seldom performed today.

Trauma

Direct blunt trauma can lead to degenerative changes in articular cartilage, but no study has determined the threshold of trauma applied to the front of the knee required to cause lasting damage to the patellofemoral cartilage.

Articular fractures of the patella and trochlea, on the other hand, can be expected to pose the same risk of arthritis as other intra-articular fractures. In their 1995 study, Argenson and colleagues [24] found that trauma was the cause of the arthritis in 20 of 66 patients who were candidates for a patellofemoral arthroplasty.

Traumatic arthritis is suited to isolated patellofemoral procedures, because the arthritis is not likely to progress rapidly to the other compartments.

Obesity

As a person climbs a staircase, gets out of a chair, or performs any other closed-chain activity, the pressures across the patellofemoral articulation increase with the person's weight. It stands to reason that obesity is a risk factor for patellofemoral arthritis. The body mass index (BMI) is the yardstick by which obesity is

Table 1
Clinical presentation of dysplasia

Dysplasia classification	Clinical presentation (%)		
	Asymptomatic arthritis	Instability + Arthritis	Instability without arthritis
No dysplasia	27	5	9
Type A	35	29	54
Type B	14	36	17
Type C	13	13	9
Type D	11	17	11

determined. The BMI is calculated as a person's weight divided by the square of the person's height. A BMI greater than 30 indicates obesity.

Obesity has been found to predispose a person to knee pain [25,26], to knee arthritis [27], and to patellofemoral arthritis [28,29].

Osteoarthritis and inflammatory arthritis

A number of patients who have seemingly isolated patellofemoral arthritis in fact suffer from osteoarthritis or inflammatory arthritis that happens to have afflicted the patellofemoral compartment first. In time, the other compartments also deteriorate. Such patients are more likely to obtain only short-term relief from a patellofemoral procedure.

Genetic components

As new causes for physical afflictions are discovered, the idiopathic category of human diseases grows smaller, and patellofemoral arthritis should be no exception. Some patients may have a genetic predisposition to deterioration of the articular cartilage. Spector and MacGregor [30], for example, have noted that the ability of collagen to withstand high stresses has a genetic component. This genetic variation probably accounts for the wide range of clinical responses to a given set of joint loads.

Summary

It behooves the surgeon contemplating patellofemoral surgery to consider the origin of the patient's arthritis. If malalignment, instability, or trauma is at the root of the problem, the surgeon can feel more confident that patellofemoral surgery will have lasting results.

References

[1] Mow VC, Hayes WC. Basic orthopaedic biomechanics. 3rd edition. New York: Lippincott Raven; 2004.
[2] Mow VC, Kuei SC, Lai WM, et al. Biphasic creep and stress relaxation of articular cartilage in compression? Theory and experiments. J Biomech Eng 1980;102(1):73–84.
[3] Ateshian GA, Hung CT. Patellofemoral joint biomechanics and tissue engineering. Clin Orthop Relat Res 2005;436:81–90.
[4] Merchant AC, Mercer RL. Lateral release of the patella. A preliminary report. Clin Orthop 1974; 139(103):40–5.
[5] Ficat P, Ficat C, Bailleux A. [External hypertension syndrome of the patella. Its significance in the recognition of arthrosis]. Rev Chir Orthop Reparatrice Appar Mot 1975;61(1):39–59 [in French].
[6] Putz R, Muller-Gerbl M, Eckstein F, et al. Are there any correlations between superficial cartilaginous alterations and subchondral bone density (CT-OAM) in the patellofemoral joint? Orthopedic Transactions 1991;15:497.
[7] Eckstein F, Muller-Gerbl M, Putz R. [The distribution of cartilage degeneration of the human patella in relation to individual subchondral mineralization]. Z Orthop Ihre Grenzgeb 1994;132(5):405–11 [in German].
[8] Iwano T, Kurosawa H, Tokuyama H, et al. Roentgenographic and clinical findings of patellofemoral osteoarthrosis. With special reference to its relationship to femorotibial osteoarthrosis and etiologic factors. Clin Orthop Relat Res 1990;252:190–7.
[9] Goutallier D, Bernageau J. Le point sur la TA-GT. In: Goutallier D, editor. La pathologie femoro-patellaire, vol. 71. Paris: Expansion Scientifique Publications; 1999. p. 175–82.
[10] Grelsamer RP, Meadows S. The modified Insall-Salvati ratio for assessment of patellar height. Clin Orthop Relat Res 1992;282:170–6.
[11] Dejour H, Walch G, Nove-Josserand L, et al. Factors of patellar instability: an anatomic radiographic study. Knee Surg Sports Traumatol Arthrosc 1994; 2(1):19–26.
[12] Dejour D, Le Coultre B. Osteotomies in patellofemoral instabilities. Sports Med Arthrosc 2007; 15(1):39–46.
[13] Grelsamer R, Weinstein C. The biomechanics of the patellofemoral joint. Clin Orthop Relat Res 2001; 389:9–14.
[14] Kwak SD, Colman WW, Ateshian GA, et al. Anatomy of the human patellofemoral joint articular cartilage: surface curvature analysis. J Orthop Res 1997;15(3):468–72.
[15] Dejour D, Allain J. Histoire naturelle de l'arthrose fémoro-patellaire isolée. Rev Chir Orthop 2004; 90(Suppl 5):1S69–129.
[16] Tavernier T, Dejour D. [Knee imaging: what is the best modality]. J Radiol 2001;82(3 Pt 2):387–405 07–8 [in French].
[17] Grelsamer RP, Tedder JL. The lateral trochlear sign. Femoral trochlear dysplasia as seen on a lateral view roentgenograph. Clin Orthop Relat Res 1992;281: 159–62.
[18] Tecklenburg K, Dejour D, Hoser C, et al. Bony and cartilaginous anatomy of the patellofemoral joint. Knee Surg Sports Traumatol Arthrosc 2006;14(3): 235–40.
[19] Caton J, Deschamps G, Chambat P, et al. [Patella infera. Apropos of 128 cases]. Rev Chir Orthop

Reparatrice Appar Mot 1982;68(5):317–25 [in French].

[20] Dejour H, Walch G, Neyret P, et al. La dysplasie de la trochlée fémorale. Rev Chir Orthop 1990;76:45–54.

[21] Maenpaa H, Lehto MU. Patellar dislocation. The long-term results of nonoperative management in 100 patients. Am J Sports Med 1997;25(2):213–7.

[22] Maenpaa H, Lehto MU. Patellofemoral osteoarthritis after patellar dislocation. Clin Orthop Relat Res 1997;339:156–62.

[23] Nikku R, Nietosvaara Y, Kallio PE, et al. Operative versus closed treatment of primary dislocation of the patella. Similar 2-year results in 125 randomized patients. Acta Orthop Scand 1997;68(5):419–23.

[24] Argenson JN, Guillaume JM, Aubaniac JM. Is there a place for patellofemoral arthroplasty? Clin Orthop Relat Res 1995;321:162–7.

[25] Andersen RE, Crespo CJ, Bartlett SJ, et al. Relationship between body weight gain and significant knee, hip, and back pain in older Americans. Obes Res 2003;11(10):1159–62.

[26] Webb R, Brammah T, Lunt M, et al. Opportunities for prevention of 'clinically significant' knee pain: results from a population-based cross sectional survey. J Public Health (Oxf) 2004;26(3):277–84.

[27] Dawson J, Juszczak E, Thorogood M, et al. An investigation of risk factors for symptomatic osteoarthritis of the knee in women using a life course approach. J Epidemiol Community Health 2003; 57(10):823–30.

[28] Cooper C, McAlindon T, Snow S, et al. Mechanical and constitutional risk factors for symptomatic knee osteoarthritis: differences between medial tibiofemoral and patellofemoral disease. J Rheumatol 1994;21(2):307–13.

[29] McAlindon T, Zhang Y, Hannan M, et al. Are risk factors for patellofemoral and tibiofemoral knee osteoarthritis different? J Rheumatol 1996;23(2): 332–7.

[30] Spector TD, MacGregor AJ. Risk factors for osteoarthritis: genetics. Osteoarthr Cartil 2004;12(Suppl A): S39–44.

Prescribing Quality Patellofemoral Rehabilitation Before Advocating Operative Care

Anil Bhave, PT[a,b],*, Erin Baker, MPT, PT[c]

[a]Rubin Institute for Advanced Orthopedics, 2401 West Belvedere Avenue, Sinai Hospital, Baltimore, MD 21215, USA
[b]Department of Physical Therapy, University of Maryland, 100 Penn Street, Baltimore, MD 21201, USA
[c]Outpatient Physical Therapy, Rubin Institute for Advanced Orthopedics Sinai Hospital, 2401 West Belvedere Avenue, Sinai Hospital, Baltimore, MD 21215, USA

In this article we discuss causes of patellofemoral dysfunction (Table 1), the treatment algorithm of nonsurgical therapy modalities, and what constitutes a quality rehabilitation protocol for a patient with patellofemoral dysfunction. We also discuss how to avoid patellofemoral problems after surgery of the knee joint. Patellofemoral pain is one of the most prevalent knee problems, affecting nearly 25% of the general population [1]. The prevalence of isolated patellofemoral arthritis may be as high as nearly 10% of patients who have painful knees [2]. The articular cartilage of the patella is the thickest in the human body and receives and distributes the most force, cushioning the joint from excessive impact. Its solid component is made of collagen and glycosaminoglycans, which encase the fluid component whose pressure provides the cushioning effect. When wear and tear produces cracks and fissures in the solid, the pressure in the fluid decreases, and the collagen bears most of the force. The ability of the collagen to withstand such forces is determined greatly by genetics, contributing to the varied presentation and mixed results from the treatment of patellofemoral pain [3]. A detailed radiographic and clinical examination is necessary to help determine what conservative measures may be most effective. About 70% of patellofemoral disorders improve with time and nonoperative management [4]. Once it is determined that the patient would benefit from conservative treatment, a well written, detailed prescription for physical therapy is needed to ensure the most appropriate care. Although strengthening, range of motion, and taping are used in the management of patellofemoral joint pain, often more specific information, such as range of motion restrictions, degree of lesion, and location of lesion, is needed to effectively treat patients.

Overall approach

We recommend that patients be classified in three categories of pain level: acute, subacute, or chronic. Patients in the subacute and chronic phases are usually considered as one group, with the chronic patient being less restricted and allowed to do a more aggressive regimen. All rehabilitation protocols are geared to fit the pain profile of the patient. Patellofemoral pain in the acute phase can be due to the initial inflammatory response after blunt trauma to the knee or a recent episode of patellar subluxation or dislocation. The patient may complain of intolerance to full-range movement, painful weight bearing, and tenderness to palpation along the medial side of the patella. The priority of conservative management in these patients is the reduction of pain and inflammation. This type of patient is fitted with a knee immobilizer or a hinged knee brace locked in full extension and is provided with pain management modalities. The use of a knee immobilizer is the

* Corresponding author. Rubin Institute for Advanced Orthopedics, 2401 West Belvedere Avenue, Sinai Hospital, Baltimore, MD 21215.
E-mail address: abhave@lifebridgehealth.org (A. Bhave).

Table 1
Static and dynamic and systemic causes of patello femoral dysfunction

Tightness or contracture	Skeletal deformation	Muscle weakness[a]/laxity	Systemic causes
Patellar tendon	Abnormal slope trochlea	Vastus medialis obliqus[a]	Obesity
Quadriceps tendon	Trochlear dysplasia	Gluteus medius[a]	Genetic predisposition
Lateral retinaculum	Malrotated trochlea	Hip flexor[a]	Occupational and sports specific
Distal ilio tibial band	Genu valgus	Hip external rotator[a]	Inflammatory diseases
Vastus lateralis	Femoral and tibial malrotation	Ankle plantar flexor[a]	High-impact torsional loads
Hamstrings	Knee flexion deformity	MPFL or LPFL laxity	
Gastrocnemius	Flatfoot (plano valgus foot)	Abnormal VMO/VL activity	
Rectus femoris			
Ilio psoas and hip adductor			

Abbreviations: a, muscle; LPFL, lateral patellofemoral ligament; MPFL, medial patellofemoral ligament; VL, vastus lateralis; VMO, vastus medialis obliquus.

least desirable option due to a lack of customization of fit, which allows for too much movement, causing continued pain and inflammation. Better options are hinged locking braces set in full extension and the use of a crescent-shaped piece of foam placed on the lateral aspect of the knee held in place with an ace wrap to promote medialization [4]. One could also use a taping protocol for stabilization of the patella with the hinged knee brace locked in full extension. To reduce strength losses while the patient's knee is immobilized, early use of quad sets is prudent to eradicate the effects of disuse atrophy and neural inhibition due to pain and swelling. Combining exercise with neuromuscular electric stimulation (NMES) enhances the positive effects of strengthening exercises [5]. NMES bypasses the reflexive neural inhibition caused by pain and effusion of the joint. As little as 20 to 30 mL of fluid has been shown to significantly decrease the H-reflex [6], a measure of motor neuron pool recruitment or excitability of the quadriceps, in the vastus medialis obliquus (VMO). It takes double that amount of knee effusion for the vastus lateralis (VL) to be inhibited (50–60 mL). This shows that VMO is far more susceptible to atrophy due to joint effusion than the VL [6]. Neural inhibition of VMO leads to decreased fiber recruitment, which causes atrophy. This leads to decreased stability about the patellofemoral joint and causes an imbalance between VMO and VL activation and contraction, leading to lateral instability of the patella. Transcutaneous nerve stimulation may be used for reduction of pain and can be used in conjunction with NMES. Cryotherapy is beneficial for reducing joint swelling and pain and for reducing muscle atrophy. It is recommended that a patient in this phase use ice therapy for as long as 6 hours every 24 hours.

A patient who has subacute or chronic joint pain may present with tolerance of movement through a small range of open-chain knee motion, partial weight bearing, and improved tolerance to palpation of surrounding knee structures. When prescribing quality physical therapy for this individual, detailed information from radiographic findings may be helpful to the therapist, specifically the location of chondral lesion (superior, central, or inferior) and whether it is full thickness or partial thickness with cartilaginous softening. This information helps the clinician to determine the exercise prescription for the patient and to shape the expectations for outcomes of therapy.

Once it is determined that the patient can be mobilized, therapy can focus on range of motion of the knee, hip, and ankle. Patellofemoral pain can be linked with tightness of numerous soft tissue structures, and mobilizations of such structures should be included in the prescription. Mobilization of the patella and flexibility of the lateral retinaculum are of primary importance. Attention should be given to improved flexibility of the distal iliotibial (IT) band, hamstring, and gastrocnemius muscles. After establishing adequate flexibility, it is important to gradually strengthen the quadriceps, hamstrings, and hip abductor muscles. It is typical to progress patients from small–arc, closed-chain resistance to a larger arc followed by open-chain exercise (Box 1). As the patient obtains adequate strength, attention is given to proprioception enhancement activities, such as balancing on a wobble board.

Box 1. Recommended progression quadriceps strengthening for pain-free resistive exercise

- Isometrics in full extension of the knee
- Straight leg raise in 30° of external rotation
- Terminal knee extension in closed chain with Theraband
- Terminal knee extension in open chain 0° to 30°
- Terminal knee extension in open chain 0° to 50°
- Terminal knee extension leg press 0° to 50°
- Shallow bilateral squat with ball between knees
- Step-up and step-down with affected limb
- Isokinetic strengthening in concentric mode high speed (210) to low speed (60)
- Reactive eccentrics low speed to high speed

Recommended additional muscle strengthening techniques
- Hip abductor strengthening
1 Side lying with ankle weight, pattern specific for gluteus medius and minimus
2 Hip hikes on a platform
3 Open chain opposite limb abduction, standing on foam
- Hip flexor and rotator
1 Resisted hip flexion with 45° inclined sitting
- Proprioceptive neuromuscular facilitation techniques
- Ankle plantarflexor
1 Open chain strengthening using Theraband
2 Closed chain with bilateral heel raise to unilateral heel raise
- Abnormal VMO/VL activity
1 Lateral to medial McConnel taping
2 EMG biofeedback

Soft tissue flexibility considerations

Some of the tight structures (Box 2) encountered in the treatment of patellofemoral disorders include a tight tensor fascia latae (TFL) with a tight IT band, leading to lateral retinaculum tightness and increased lateral pull on the patella. Addressing this starts with a modified Ober stretch for the TFL (Fig. 1) followed by deep friction massage (DFM) along the IT band and down to the distal aspect where it feeds into the lateral retinaculum. DFM facilitates a breakdown of

Box 2. Recommended mobilization and stretching

- Patellar and quad tendon
  DFM
  Tape (kinesio)
- Lateral retinaculum
  DFM
  McConnell tape
  Distal IT and VL stretch
- Distal IT band
  DFM
  Modified Ober position with the knee at 30° of flexion and knee joint varus mobilization
- Hamstrings
  Straight leg raise with opposite limb immobilized, internal rotation at the hip for localized stretch on medial hamstring and external rotation for biceps
- Gastrocnemius
  Closed-chain standing stretch in slight internal rotation
- Rectus femoris
  Ely test position in prone or sidelying
- Iliopsoas
  Thomas test or Kendall position
- Hip adductor
  Stretch in hip flexion and extension

Secondary Rx considerations
  Weight shifts using balance platforms
  Bilateral squats on foam
  Limb perturbation in standing on tilt board
  Unilateral squats on foam
  Foot orthotics
  Activity modification
  Ergonomic and postural training

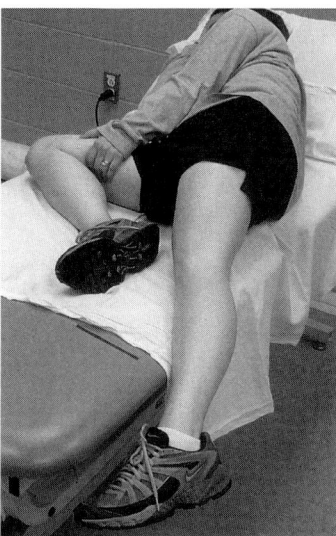

Fig. 1. Self-stretch in the Ober position of the TFL and ITB. The patient is in sidelying with the affected limb up and pulls the unaffected bottom limb to the chest for pelvic stabilization. The patient then extends the affected limb off the bed and externally rotates the hip before letting gravity pull the limb into adduction to provide the stretch.

adhesions with the overlying fascia [7], helps in mobilization of the IT band, and improves patellar tracking. With the patient in the modified Ober position, the therapist can apply a varus force on the distal tibia with the knee flexed about 30° for additional distal IT band stretching. The use of McConnell taping [8] for medialization of the patella provides a prolonged stretch to the tissues of the lateral retinaculum and allows for better patellar positioning and pain relief.

Hamstring tightness results in a knee flexion contracture. This limits the ability of the patellafemoral joint to be unloaded through knee extension, thus causing increased compression and pain. A flexed knee joint is subjected to greater patellofemoral compressive forces than in a fully extended knee. Therefore, hamstring stretching is necessary in a comprehensive rehabilitation program. It is recommended that medial hamstrings be stretched in internal rotation of the hip and lateral hamstrings be stretched in external rotation. Rotation of the hip during a hamstring stretch maximizes the effectiveness of the stretch (Fig. 2). Knee flexion contracture (Fig. 3) is not only the product of tight hamstrings but also can result from a tight gastrocnemius muscle, a tight capsule, and tight hip flexor muscles (iliopsoas and rectus femoris). Patients who have a tight gastrocnemius muscle may attempt to walk with a plantigrade ankle, forcing their knee into flexion and causing an increased patellofemoral compressive force. Typical mobilizations for the gastrocnemius are ankle dorsiflexion with full knee extension in the closed or open chain position. This position can be modified by flexing the knee to stretch the soleus. Tightness in the hip flexors may seem to be a knee flexion contracture when the patient is in the supine position. If the hip flexors are tight, then the knee flexion contracture reduces or resolves in the long sit position. In our clinical experience, we have found two excellent ways to stretch the hip flexors: via the Thomas test position or the Kendall position (Fig. 4). Both positions provide better lumbo-pelvic stabilization than simple prone lying for the stretching of the iliopsoas. The Thomas test position and the Kendall positions can be used in conjunction with knee flexion to stretch the rectus femoris muscle. Tyler and colleagues [9] found that positive Thomas and Ober tests were significant in patients who have patellofemoral pain. These abnormalities cause anterior pelvic tilt with internal rotation of the femur during function. Internal rotation of the femur results in lateral tracking of the patella in the trochlea. This leads to increased patellofemoral compressive forces, which may contribute to pain and eventual patellofemoral arthritis. Therefore, stretching the hip flexors and Tensor Fascia Lata is a vital addition to the physical therapy prescription [9]. It is important to also pay attention to Rectus femoris tightness as tested in Ely position (Fig. 5) and to palpate for tightness of the quadriceps tendon and lateral retinaculum. Tightness of these structures causes superior tracking of the patella during knee flexion. This leads to excessive stretch and compressive force on the patellar tendon, leading to anterior knee pain. Deep friction massage to these structures and pulsed ultrasound improve flexibility.

Muscle strength considerations

Recommending strengthening exercises for the musculature around the knee joint is a critical component of patellofemoral rehabilitation. The notion of working through pain is not a prudent concept for a patient suffering from patellofemoral pain. Knee joint effusion causes atrophy of the extensor mechanism of the knee and inhibits

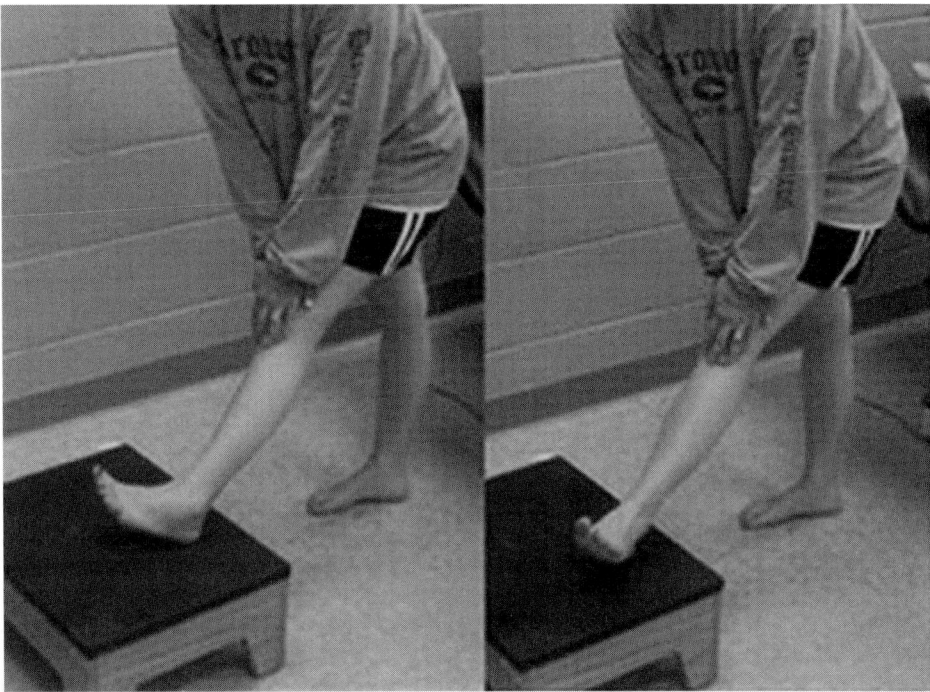

Fig. 2. A self-stretching technique where the patient places the heel on a step and with knee extended and reaches toward the toes to stretch the hamstrings. Internal rotation focuses the stretch on the lateral hamstrings, and external rotation focuses the stretch on the medial hamstrings.

quadriceps force production [6,10], but allowing aggressive strengthening too soon can be detrimental to the success of the rehabilitation program. Dye [11] recommended that the therapist must keep activities within the available envelope of function for healing and homeostasis to occur.

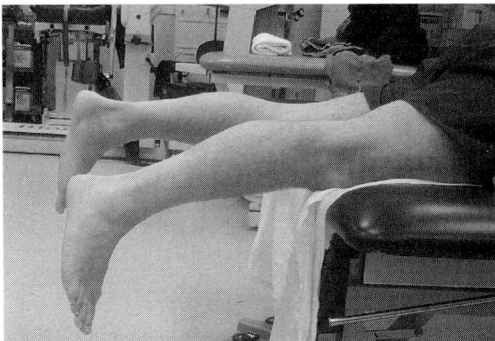

Fig. 3. Self-stretch into knee extension where the patient lies in the prone position and allows gravity to pull the lower leg down into extension to stretch the hamstrings. Progression of the stretch involves applying weights to the distal tibia.

It is important to start with submaximal, pain-free activities and to avoid activities that cause inflammation of the patellofemoral joint. Open- and closed-chain exercise can be beneficial, but it must be understood when each type of exercise is appropriate. Escamilla and colleagues [12] noted that quadriceps activity is greatest in closed chain near full flexion and in open chain near full extension. Open chain produces more rectus femoris activity, and closed chain promotes vasti activity. Patellofemoral compressive forces are greatest in closed-chain activity near full flexion and are greatest in mid-range of knee extension with open chain activity. With this information, a comprehensive and logical pain-free exercise program can be prescribed. In the acute phase of patellofemoral pain, movement should be avoided, and isometric exercise should be prescribed. Once the patient is in the subacute phase, an increase in movement from extension to flexion can be progressed, and a progression from open-chain to closed-chain exercise is recommended (see Box 2). The ideal progression from isometrics starts with straight leg raises and can be combined with external rotation to recruit more fibers from

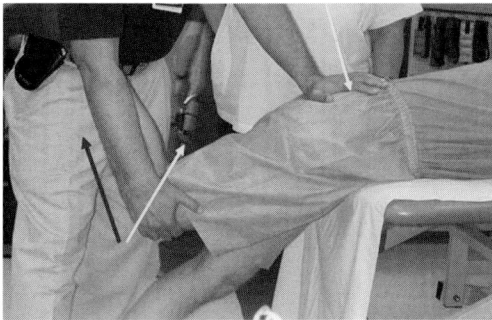

Fig. 4. The Kendall position is used to stretch the hip flexors and the TFL. With the pelvis stabilized into the mat, the limb is brought into extension (for the hip flexors) and slight adduction (for the TFL) and held at the point where resistance is felt or the pelvis starts to anteriorly tilt.

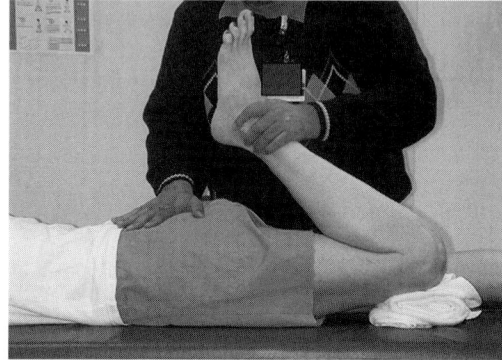

Fig. 5. Prone knee flexion mobilization with pelvic stabilization over the ipsilateral posterior superior iliac spine for stretching the rectus femoris.

the medial quads and specifically the VMO. Next, open-chain knee extension is appropriate within 0° to 30° (short arc), staying out of the mid-range knee motion where patellofemoral compressive forces are greatest. The patient can progress to open-chain knee extension from 0° to 50°, provided it is through pain-free range. Thomee [13] allowed activities with up to 5/10 pain on a visual analogue scale, provided the pain dissipated immediately once the exercise terminated. However,

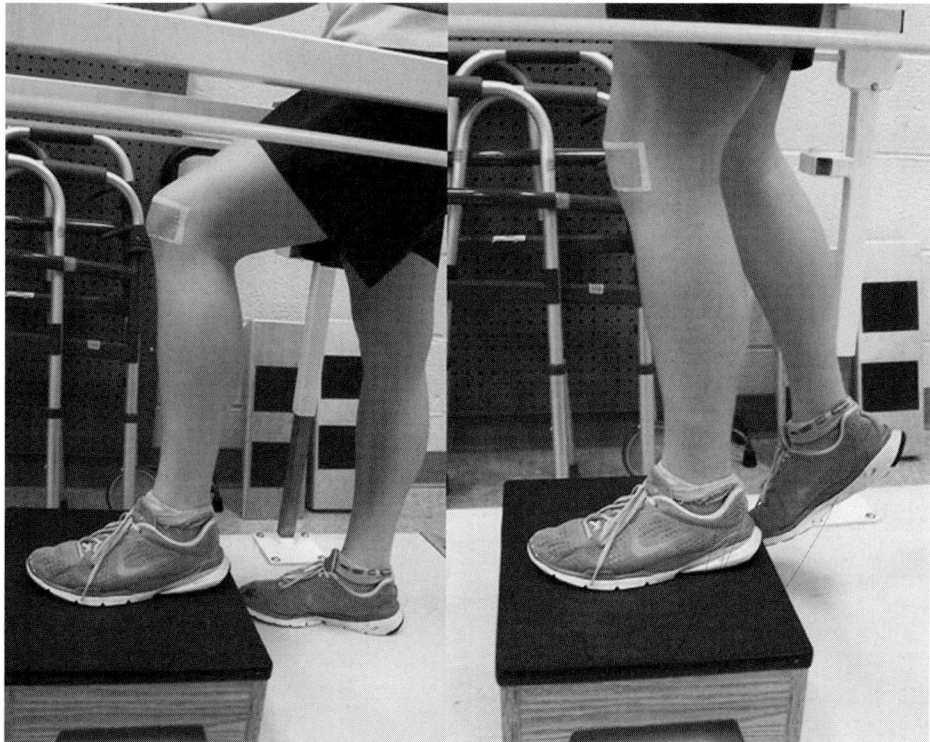

Fig. 6. Step-up exercise for closed-chain quadriceps strengthening using McConnell tape to prevent lateral displacement of the patella during knee flexion and extension.

the gold standard in patellofemoral rehabilitation is identifying a pain-free range of the motion during therapeutic exercise. After 0° to 50° open-chain exercise is tolerated, the patient should be progressed to closed-chain exercise on the leg press 0° to 50° followed by shallow double leg squats. Next in the progression are step-up and step-down activities (Fig. 6), starting with a small step (6–8 inches) and progressing to larger steps (8–14 inches) because larger steps lead to higher compressive forces at the patellofemoral joint from increased closed-chain knee flexion. One of the last exercises a patient who has patellofemoral pain can tolerate is concentric and eccentric isokinetic exercise in open chain starting at high speeds in concentric mode with a progression of decreased speed and then eccentric mode with higher speeds for increasing control. We advocate the use of taping (Fig. 7) during advancement of strengthening exercise as a protective measure with more provocative tasks.

A proper prescription outlines range of motion restrictions per phase of healing (acute, subacute, or chronic) and whether the lesion is distal or proximal on the patella. Deep knee flexion exercises are avoided for proximal lesions, and early flexion should be avoided for distal lesions. If the lesion involves full-thickness loss of the articular cartilage (ie, patellofemoral arthritis [3]), the patient must be instructed to modify the activity and avoid the parts of the range where the compressive forces are greatest. Central lesions are most difficult because compressive forces are greatest through greater ranges of motion at mid-range and at flexion past 90° [3].

The use of NMES to the quadriceps muscle should be prescribed for patients who have patellofemoral pain. Stevens and colleagues [5] showed that patients who undergo maximal isometric quadriceps contractions elicited by NMES as part of their rehabilitation programs showed greater strength in the affected leg after 6 months when compared with the unaffected leg. Patents who did not use NMES were weaker in their affected limb at 6 months. The use of NMES with the prescribed exercise program expedites strengthening of the quadriceps mechanism and increases the stability of the patellofemoral joint. The key in quadriceps strengthening exercises is to apply a supramaximal stimulation and augment voluntary contraction by a superimposed electrical stimulation. This type of stimulation can be combined with all of the quadriceps strengthening activities (see Box 2).

Emphasis has been given to quadriceps strengthening exercises; however, it is also important to address hip joint strength in these patients. Weakness of the hip flexor causes anterior pelvic tilt with internal rotation of the femur during function due to lack of eccentric control. Internal rotation of the femur results in lateral tracking of the patella in the trochlea. This leads to increased patellofemoral compressive forces, which may contribute to pain and eventual patellofemoral arthritis. Therefore, hip flexor strengthening is recommended.

Another muscle that needs attention is the gluteus medius. Cichanowski and colleagues [14] assessed hip strength in female collegiate athletes who had unilateral symptoms of patellofemoral pain. The study showed statistically significant correlation between hip abductor and external rotator weakness and patellofemoral pain. Weakness of the hip abductors and external rotators allows the femur to internally rotate during closed-chain activities. This leads to an apparent valgus in the knee, causing maltracking of the patella and a resultant lateral contact of the patella

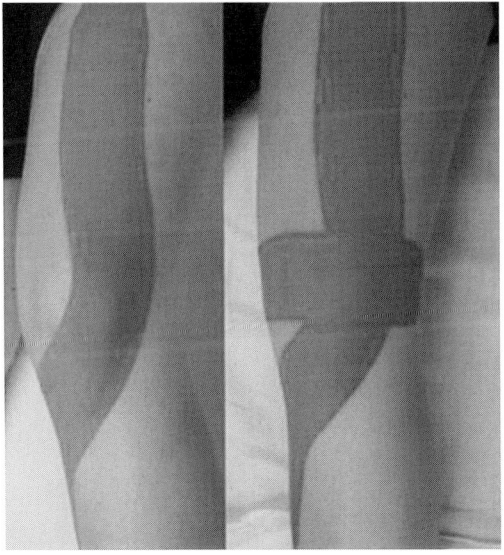

Fig. 7. A patellar taping technique using Kinesiotape. The first piece is placed over the rectus femoris and comes down to the lateral aspect of the patella and is pulled over to the medial aspect of the tibia to provide a patellar cradle and promote proper patellar inferior translation during knee flexion and extension. A second piece of tape is placed directly lateral to the patella and pulled medially with 50% tension to emphasize medial translation of the patella and to hold it in the femoral trochlea during movement.

in the trochlea. As far as the hip musculature is concerned, loss of eccentric control of the hip flexors and weakness of the abductors and external rotators leads to internal rotation (Fig. 8) of the femur in closed-chain and thus patellar maltracking and pain. Hip abductors and rotators can be strengthened in open chain with weights at the ankle. It is also important to facilitate hip muscles in closed chain through activities such as step-ups and using a wobble board or balance master (see Fig. 8).

Role of taping

In our clinical experience, the use of patellar taping techniques has been beneficial for prolonged soft tissue stretch. Studies have explored the proper technique for its use and the true physiologic effects it has on the patellofemoral joint and surrounding structures. Gilleard and colleagues [15] found in a controlled study of taping versus nontaping that patellar taping was associated with earlier firing of the vastus medialis obliquus (VMO) than the VL in closed-chain step-up and step-down activities. Cowan and colleagues [16] found the same results and compared patellofemoral taping with placebo tape and and found that only the patellofemoral taping caused the timing of the VMO to be sooner in the stair stepping activities. Both studies give credence to the use of patellar taping in improving the timing of the VMO to provide medial stabilization of the patella during provocative tasks.

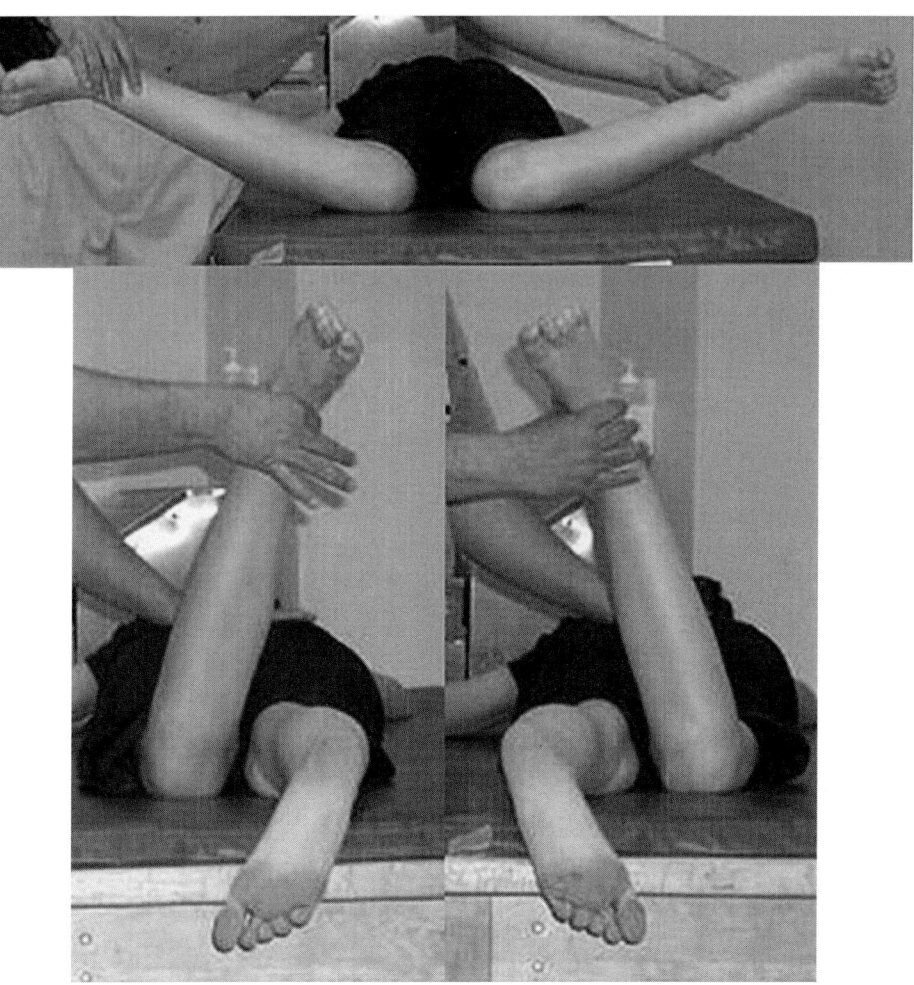

Fig. 8. Careful hip rotation measurement.

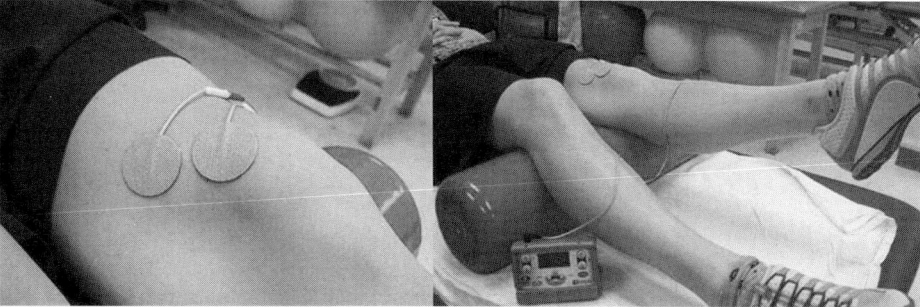

Fig. 9. NMES is applied to the oblique fibers of the vastus medialis, which recent cadaver dissections have shown the VMO to have its own innervation. It is theorized that using NMES on the oblique fibers may change the force vector of the vastus medialis as a whole, thereby improving the control of the patella in the trochlear groove.

The function of the VMO and its relevance to patellofemoral joint pain have been disputed in the literature. Toumi and colleagues [17] investigated the function of the VMO compared with the VL using surface EMG and found that the VMO was more active at knee angles where the patella was less stable in the trochlear groove (angles closer to full extension) during jumping activities; it was concluded that the VMO is a patellar stabilizer rather than a muscle that moves the patella medially. In this study, the VMO was active even when the subjects were in the air from a jump, further indicating the role of stabilization. Applying such information to the clinic may give supporting argument to the efficacy of patellar taping for medialization to improve the length–tension relationship of the VMO and thus stimulate quicker firing during stepping activities presumably resulting in increased patella stabilization. Through cadaveric dissection, Toumi [17] also found that the VMO had attachments not only to the patellar tendon but also attached directly to the medial border of the patella, allowing it to better influence the movement of the patella. It was noted to have its own innervation separate from the innervation to the proximal vastus medialis. We hypothesize that if neuromuscular electrical stimulation is applied to the VMO (Fig. 9) and the contractile capabilities are improved, the force vector of the vastus medialis as a whole may be changed to provide the patella with more medial stability and decrease the pain around the joint. Taping to medialize the patella remains one of the hallmarks of patellofemoral rehabilitation. We recommend taping for VMO activation for potential stabilization during rehabilitation and during functional activities and during sports. A clinical guideline of 50% reduction in pain after taping for activities such as step-ups or resistive open- or closed-chain exercises is recommended and should be the goal of taping. It is our practice to tape the patella before exercise to promote better alignment and to balance the forces around the patella before it moves into the trochlea during knee flexion. If the patella is not taped, there is a risk of promoting further lateralization of the patella because the VMO will not be able to stabilize the patella and the medial retinaculum will be stretched. It is our goal to use taping to control

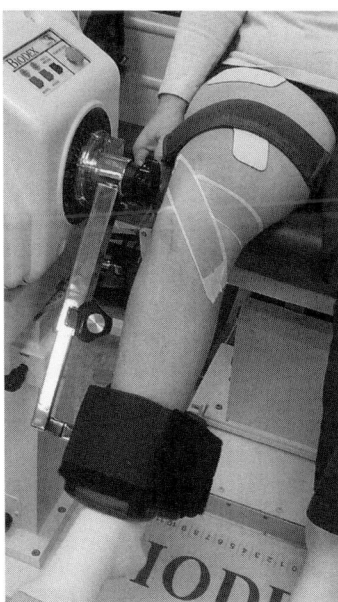

Fig. 10. E-stim with isometrics using protocol from Stevens and colleagues [5] for end-range knee extension strengthening. Proper patellar position within the femoral trochlea is emphasized using McConnell taping.

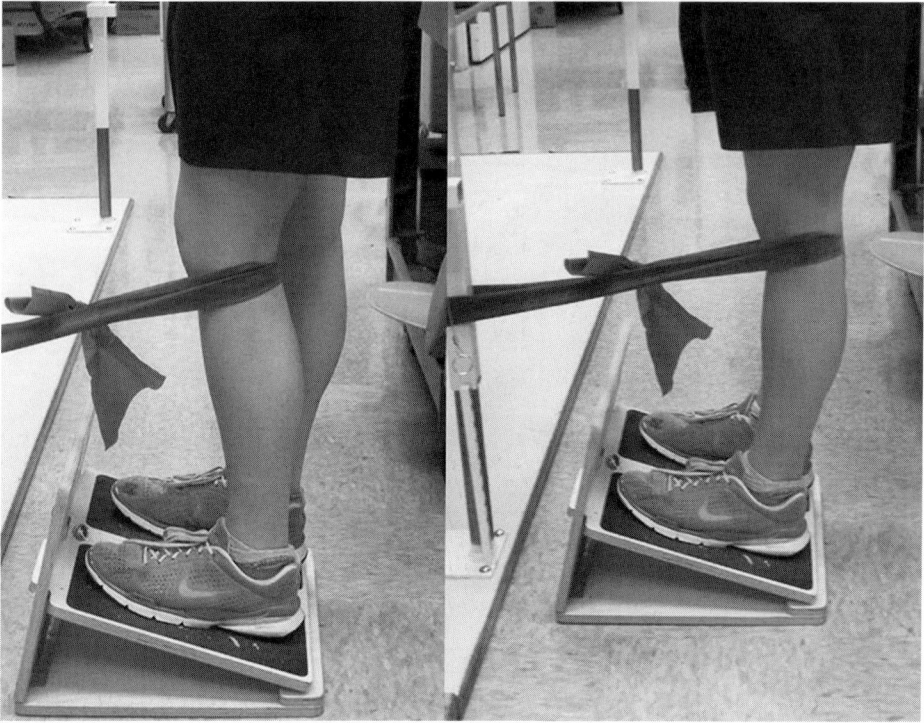

Fig. 11. Closed-chain quadriceps strengthening. Terminal knee extension exercise using a Therabandfor resistance in the closed chain position to strengthen and mobilize into end-range knee extension.

patellar glide, tilt, and malrotation. The use of taping throughout rehabilitation to promote VMO activation and avoid maltracking of the patella is the hallmark of patellofemoral rehabilitation. One of the newer techniques available to therapists is Kinesiotape (Kinesio USA, Albuquerque, NM). This is more flexible tape and allows greater freedom of motion, especially in athletic activity. Kinesiotape can be used to facilitate VMO, control patellar glide or tilt, and inhibit excessive VL firing. More research is needed on this to prove the efficacy of this technique.

Summary

Patellofemoral pain is difficult to treat. Several skeletal deformities are risk factors, such as increased q angle, flatfeet, femoral anteversion, patellar or femoral dysplasia, and atrophy of VMO. In the acute phase, the goal of therapy is to reduce inflammation, increase patellar mobility, and improve quadriceps strength. The use of ice and NMES are particularly useful modalities early on. If lateral structures are tight, then gentle DFM and pulsed ultrasound are useful to break up scar tissue and improve flexibility. The use of taping to stabilize patellar glide and tilt is also useful. Gradual strengthening beginning from isometrics and straight leg raises to resisted short arc quads can then be performed. Therapist must follow the principles advocated by Dye [11] of submaximal pain-free exercise and work within the available envelope of function for healing and homeostasis. In subacute and chronic phases, the goal is to have minimal inflammation and pain mostly on provocative activities, such as deep knee bends or high step-ups. Goals of therapy include normalization of patellar mobility and improved flexibility of tight muscles around the knee and hip joint. Improved tracking of the patella, initially with the aid of taping, and improved strength and control of the quadriceps muscle are also goals. One must also include improved proprioception and neuromuscular control in closed chain. If progression to greater loads is not possible, the therapist must evaluate the taping technique and correct all components of maltracking of the patella including glide, tilt, and rotation.

Taping allows for greater load tolerance, and more challenging tasks during therapy can be achieved. The progression of quad strengthening without causing retopatellar sharp pain is also critical. The therapist should only allow generalized muscle pain during exercise and avoid joint compressive pain. Muscle stretching and restoration of patellar mobility should be achieved before progressing too far in to strengthening exercise. VMO strengthening and electrical stimulation (Fig. 10) during quadriceps strengthening are hallmarks of patellofemoral rehabilitation. In addition, improved eccentric control of the hip flexors and strength of the hip abductors and adductors are critical to correct rotation of the femur during closed-chain activities (Fig. 11) and should be emphasized. Once strength has begun to improve and range of motion is restored, additional closed-chain proprioceptive enhancement exercises, such as a wobble board, allow the patient to return to function. Careful regular follow-up and modification of home exercise program allows the patient to function well. By following these guidelines, the majority of patients (70%) will get better and return to full function.

References

[1] DeHaven KE, Lintner DM. Athletic injuries: comparison by age, sport, and gender. Am J Sports Med 1986;14(3):218–24.

[2] Davies A, Vince A, Shepstone L, et al. The radiologic prevalence of patellofemoral osteoarthritis. Clin Orthop Relat Res 2002;402:206–12.

[3] Grelsamer R, Ronald P, Stein D, et al. Patellofemoral arthritis. J Bone Joint Surg 2006;88:1849–60.

[4] Wilk K, Reinold M. Principles of patellofemoral rehabilitation. Sports Medicine Arthroscopic Review 2001;9:325–36.

[5] Stevens J, Mizner R, Snyder-Mackler L. Neruomuscular electrical stimulation for quadriceps muscle strengthening after bilateral total knee arthroplasty: a case series. J Orthop Sports Phys Ther 2004;34:21–9.

[6] Hopkins J, Ingersoll C, Krause B, et al. Effects of knee joint effusion on quadriceps and soleus motoneuron pool excitability. Med Sci Sports Exerc 2001;33(1):123–6.

[7] Fredericson M, Powers C. Practical management of patellofemoral pain. Clin J Sport Med 2002;12:36–8.

[8] McConnell J. The management of chondromalacia patellae: a long term solution. Aust J Physiother Australian Journal of Physiotherapy 1986;32:215–23.

[9] Tyler T, Nicholas S, Mullaney M, et al. The role of hip muscle function in the treatment of patellofemoral syndrome. Am J Sports Med 2006;34(4):630–6.

[10] Thomee R, Restrom P, Karlsson J. Patellofemoral pain syndrome in young women: ii. Muscle function in patients and healthy controls. Scand J Med Sci Sports 1995;5(4):245–51.

[11] Dye S. The pathophysiology of patellofemoral pain: a tissue homeostasis perspective. Clin Orthop Relat Res 2005;436:100–10. 12.

[12] Escamilla RF, Fleisig GS, Zheng N, et al. Biomechanics of the knee during closed kinetic chain and open kinetic chain exercises. Med Sci Sports Exerc 1998;30(4):556–69. 13.

[13] Thomee R. A comprehensive treatment approach for patellofemoral pain syndrome in young women. Phys Ther 1997;77:1690–703.

[14] Cichanowski H, Schmitt J, Johnson R, et al. Hip strength in collegiate female athletes with patellofemoral pain. Med Sci Sports Exerc 2007;39(8):1227–32.

[15] Gilleard W, McConnell J, Parsons D. The effect of patellar taping on the onset of vastus medialis obliquus and vastus lateralis muscle activity in persons with patellofemoral pain. Phys Ther 1998;78:25–32.

[16] Cowan S, Bennell K, Hodges P. Therapeutic patellar taping changes the timing of vasti muscle activation in people with patellofemoral pain syndrome. Clin J Sports Med 2002;12:339–47.

[17] Toumi H, Poumarat G, Benjamin M, et al. New insights into the function of the vastus medialis with clinical implications. Med Sci Sports Exerc 2007;39:1153–9.

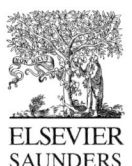

Patellofemoral Syndrome a Paradigm for Current Surgical Strategies

Robert A. Teitge, MD*

Department of Orthopaedic Surgery, Wayne State University, School of Medicine, 530 E. Canfield Street, Detroit, MI 48201, USA

Patellofemoral syndrome: What does it mean? Historically a wastebasket term for pain or dysfunction thought to come from the anterior knee, the diagnosis of patellofemoral syndrome really means we do not know what is causing the pain or the dysfunction. Often patellofemoral syndrome is not a diagnosis but rather an admission of ignorance. The literature is replete with clinical or radiological observations made in an attempt to explain and connect patellofemoral symptoms with anatomic or radiological observations. In this article, the author presents the framework used for the past 30 years to make sense of the disparate observations in the literature and to facilitate practical evaluation of the patient with the syndrome of pain or dysfunction in the anterior knee.

Two case examples are useful to stimulate clinical analysis. Case 1: A 42-year-old male state police officer presented with pain that limits walking to a few blocks, inhibits sitting in one position for more than 20 minutes, and prevents participation in all sport and exercise programs. Past history notes that he dislocated his patella playing college football and was treated with a medial tibial tubercle transfer. He has had no additional surgeries. Figs. 1 and 2 show his radiograph and CT. What would you do?

Case 2: A 26-year-old female presented with pain in the front of the knee. The pain has now made it difficult to continue playing softball and volleyball, which until recently she had done 5 or 6 nights a week. She has had no history of instability,

injury, or surgery. Her radiographs are shown in Fig. 3. What would you do? Additional data obtained in the workup and the recommended treatment are provided at the end of the article.

Literature review

If we search for a specific answer in the literature to "anterior knee pain," we often end up confused by conflicting or incomplete data and little direction. Such a search will likely uncover a number of overlapping and imprecise diagnoses, including anterior knee pain, patellofemoral syndrome, chondromalacia patella, patellar instability, patellofemoral arthritis, and patellar malalignment.

No fewer than 56 factors are cited in the literature as having an association with these diagnoses (Box 1). There may be others that the author missed.

The literature may leave us confused and lost. It should be obvious that many of these factors are poorly defined or measured and the evidence to support some is weak. Even our ability to conduct a physical examination has been challenged. Tomsich and colleagues [1] concluded that both clinical and instrumented measurements of quadriceps angle (Q-angle), A-angle, patellar tilt mediolateral, patellar mediolateral position, superoinferior tilt, and patellar rotation were too unreliable to be used. Greene and colleagues [2] noted poor interobserver and intraobserver reliability of Q-angle measurements and emphasized that the evaluation and treatment of a patient with patellofemoral symptoms should not be based on a quadriceps angle measurement.

It should also be obvious that many of the listed factors coexist. It should also be clear that the relative importance of one variable over another

* 3272 East 12 Mile Road, Warren, MI 48092.
E-mail address: rteitge@hotmail.com

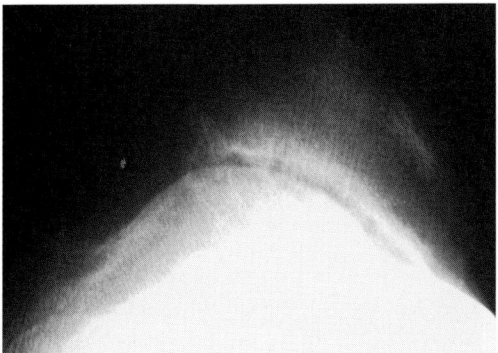

Fig. 1. Patellofemoral axial radiograph of case 1.

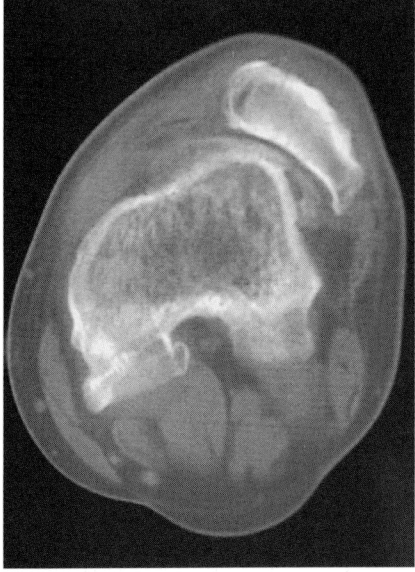

Fig. 2. CT of patellofemoral joint in 42-year-old who dislocated patella in college football and was treated at age 23 with medial transfer of tibial tubercle and lateral retinacular release (case 1).

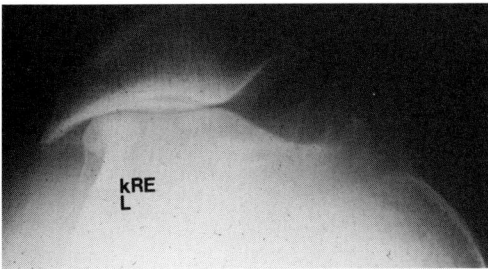

Fig. 3. Study case 2. Axial radiograph of patellofemoral joint of 28-year-old female athlete with no prior surgery or injury.

Box 1. Factors cited in the literature for association with diagnoses related to anterior knee pain

Genu valgum
Genu varum
Femoral retroversion
Femoral anteversion
Excess external tibial torsion
Outerbridge ridge
Trochlear dysplasia
Short lateral trochlea
Shallow trochlea
Increased quadriceps angle
Decreased quadriceps angle
Excess lateral quadriceps pull
Insufficient vastus medialis obliquus
Abnormal patellar spin
Patellar dysplasia
Patella alta
Patella baja
Menisectomy
Laxity or insufficiency of the anterior cruciate ligament, the posterior cruciate ligament, the lateral collateral ligament, or the medial collateral ligamentany, or of any combination of these ligaments
Rotatory instability
Iliotibial band contracture
Quadriceps contracture
Achilles' contracture
Retinacular contracture (ie, tight lateral retinaculum)
Retinacular laxity
Pes planus and hyperpronation
Abnormal distance between tibial tubercle and trochlear groove
Patellar malalignment
Patellar instability
Chondral softening
Genu recurvatum
Patellar tilt
Patellar shift
Abnormal tracking
Vastus medialis obliquus dysplasia
J-sign
A-sign
Bayonet sign
Crossing sign
Lateral patellofemoral angle
Lateral patellofemoral index

- Trochlear bump
- Patellar thickness
- Knee flexion contracture
- Ratio of vastus medialis to vastus lateralis
- Hindfoot varus
- Patellar glide
- Quadriceps tendon width
- Flexor hallucis longus dysfunction or pulley contracture
- Increased lumbar lordosis
- Increased thoracolumbar extension
- Hip flexion contracture
- Lumbopelvic instability
- Abdominal oblique muscle to psoas and rectus femoris imbalance
- Excess lateral pressure
- Female gender

has not been determined. If indeed all of these are important, then the evaluation of a patient with "patellofemoral syndrome" or its equivalent must take into consideration each of these factors.

At the root of this confusion is evidence that certain teachings handed down as dogma may have originated from incomplete readings or from illogical conclusions. For example "patellar malalignment" was defined by John Insall and colleagues [3] as being either one of two conditions: (1) an increased Q-angle or (2) a high riding patella. Insall goes on to observe:

An increased Q-angle *is usually associated* with increased femoral anteversion and external tibial torsion. In the presence of these abnormalities when the hip and ankle joints are normally aligned, the patella faces inward and motion of the knee occurs about an axis which is rotated medially compared with the axes of the hip and ankle joints.

The suggested treatment for this increased anteversion and external tibial torsion was tibial tubercle transfer. It should be of no surprise that 61% of patients remained with some persistent discomfort or instability and, in 24%, the result was unsatisfactory because the primary pathology—the medially directed knee joint axis—was not treated. However he states that if the medial tubercle transfer, which was called "patellar realignment," was combined with excision of the chondromalacic cartilage, the results were satisfactory in 79% of patients. These observations do not make sense when addressing the salient issue. Namely, what is the problem? Is the problem the increased Q-angle or the medially rotated knee-joint axis? If 61% of patients remained symptomatic after tibial tubercle transfer, why then are 79% satisfactory after medial tubercle transfer and excision of damaged cartilage? Why does just excision of damaged cartilage fail? How many patients had increased Q-angle? How many had a medially rotated knee axis? How much was it rotated? What was the actual femoral torsion? What was the actual tibial torsion? How accurate are the measures? What about a high-riding patella? Why is a high-riding patella called the second type of

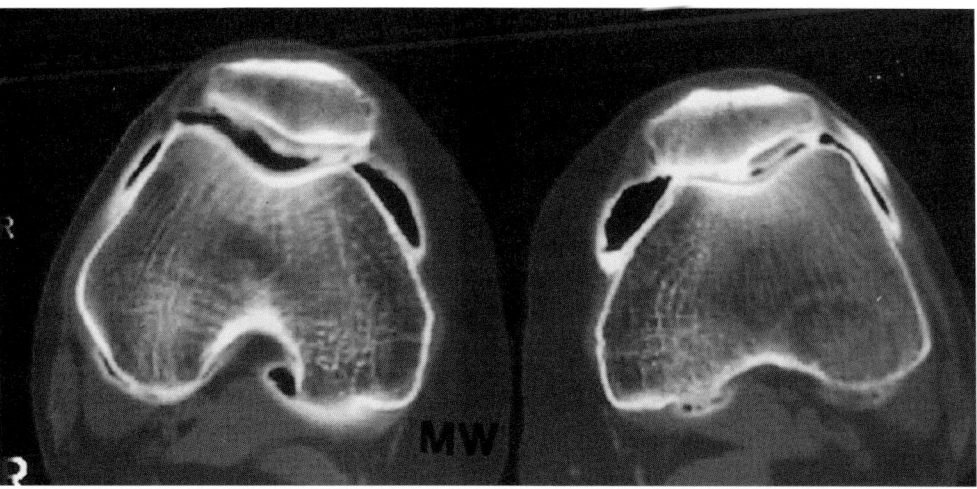

Fig. 4. CT-arthrogram of patient with bilateral medial patellofemoral joint arthritis 15 years post–bilateral medial transfer of tibial tubercle.

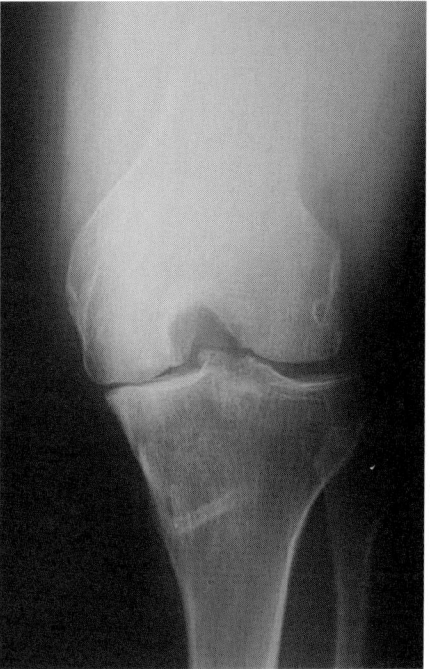

Fig. 5. Medial compartment arthritis in a patient 20 years after a medial transfer of the tibial tubercle.

patellar malalignment? Is patellar malalignment limited to an increased Q-angle or a high-riding patella? Why is a normally aligned hip and ankle joint with a medially rotated patella and knee-joint axis not a "malalignment"? A review of the literature must ask these questions if we are to understand the etiology and treatment of "anterior knee pain."

What does current scientific knowledge tell us?

Is there a consensus in literature-based evidence regarding prevalent surgical-based dogma? Current belief suggests that a medial tibial tubercle transfer with or without lateral release is somewhat of a panacea. Many clinical studies,

Table 1
Lateral facet pressure reduction

Tibial tubercle transfer	Pressure reduction
3-mm distal transfer	75%
6-mm distal transfer	52%
15-mm anterior transfer	50%
10-mm anterior + 6-mm medial transfers	20%
10-mm anterior + 6-mm lateral transfers	40%

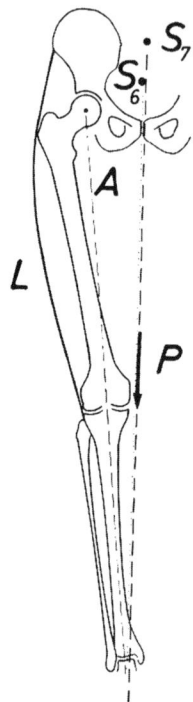

Fig. 6. The major vectors crossing the knee joint include the body weight-bearing vector (P) and the lateral muscle pull (L). A, mechanical axix; S_7, center of mass; S_6, center of mass of the whole body. (*From* Maquet PGJ. Biomechanics of the knee. Berlin: Springer-Verlag; 1976. p. 22; with permission.)

but few laboratory studies, support medial tubercle transfer. The natural history of medial tibial tubercle transfer is often medial patellofemoral joint arthrosis (Fig. 4) and then later medial compartment arthrosis (Fig. 5). Biomechanical studies would predict this clinical observation. Kuroda and colleagues [4] in the laboratory showed essentially that medial tubercle transfer overloads the medial compartment. Ostermeier and colleagues [5] have shown in the laboratory that the medial tubercle transfer had no significant effect on reducing stress on the medial patellofemoral ligament or on providing a stabilizing effect on the patella in contrast to that provided by medial patellofemoral ligament reconstruction. Thus, tubercle transfer would not be expected to be useful for the treatment of patellar instability. Huberti and Hayes [6] noted in 1984 that moving the tubercle medially increased medial facet pressure. Kelman and colleagues [7] noted that medial tubercle transfer did not pull the patella medially but rather pulled the tibia into external rotation and,

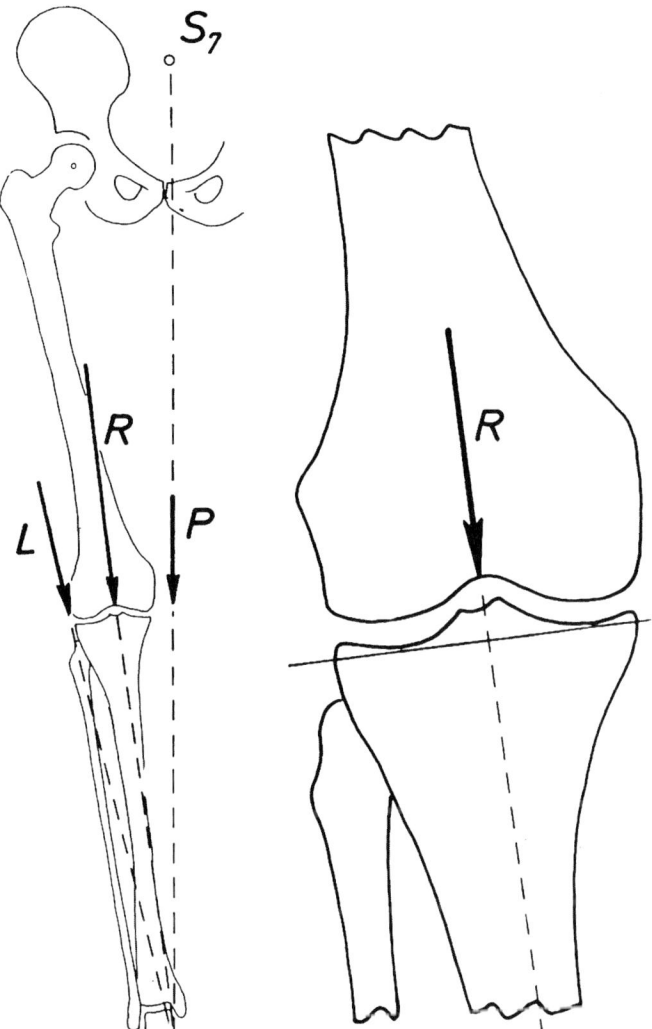

Fig. 7. The resultant vector (R) is the sum of the weight vector (P) and the lateral muscle vector (L). The resultant vector acts at the center of the knee joint and is perpendicular to the articular surface. S_7, center of mass of the entire body when standing on one foot less the mass of the limb on which one is standing. (*From* Maquet P. Osteotomy. In: Freeman MAR, Aubriot JH, editors. Arthritis of the knee. Berlin: Springer-Verlag; 1980. p. 153; with permission.)

indeed, many patients after medial tuberosity transfer walk with the foot pointed more outward. Huber and colleagues data [8] reflect unpredictability in estimating how patellofemoral contact pressures change after tubercle transfers (Table 1).

Medial transfer destroys the normal distance from the tibial tubercle to the trochlear groove, which was found by Dejour and colleagues [9] to average 14 mm in controls and which is greater than 20 mm in a high percentage of patients with objective patellar instability. Jack Hughston and Walsh [10] observed: "Asking the tubercle to control the patella is asking the tail to wag the dog."

My personal view is: Do not transfer the tibial tubercle. It evolved to be lateral for a very important biomechanical reason. The dogmas I was taught—transfer the tibial tubercle, advance the vastus medialis obliquus, or release the lateral retinaculum—are not supported by biomechanical evidence. Challenge these dogmas.

Likewise, lateral retinacular release lacks biomechanical data to support its use. Christoforakis and colleagues [11] showed that the lateral retinaculum provided up to 19% of the resistance to lateral displacement of the patella, thus suggesting that the patient having undergone lateral release is

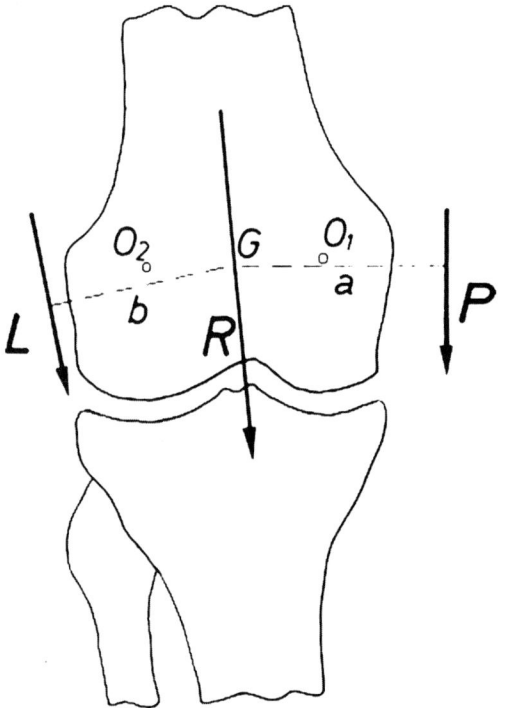

Fig. 8. Weight transmission to the ground follows the resultant vector (R) passing through the knee joint near the medial tibial spine. a, lever arm of vector P—drawn perpendicular to vector P to point G; b, lever arm of vector L—drawn perpendicular to vector L to point G; G, central point on the axis of flexion of the knee; L, lateral muscular stay; O_1, center of curvature of the medial femoral condyle; O_2, center of curvature of the lateral femoral condyle; P, weight of the part of the body supported by the knee. (*From* Maquet PGJ. Biomechanics of the knee. Berlin: Springer-Verlag; 1976. p. 23; with permission.)

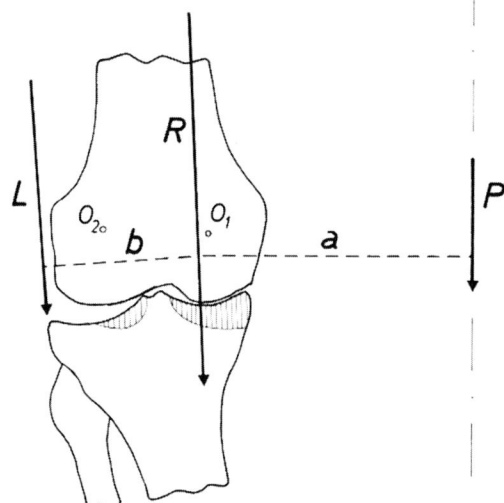

Fig. 9. If there is a reduction in the lateral muscle vector (L) or an increase in the weight vector (P), the resultant vector (R) shifts to the medial compartment, eventually resulting in medial compartment arthritis. a, lever arm of vector P—drawn perpendicular to vector P to point G; b, lever arm of vector L—drawn perpendicular to vector L to point G; O_1, center of curvature of the medial femoral condyle; O_2, center of curvature of the lateral femoral condyle. (*From* Maquet PGJ. Biomechanics of the knee. Berlin: Springer-Verlag; 1976. p. 75; with permission.)

likely to be more unstable in the lateral direction. Huberti and Hayes [12] showed that lateral release resulted in no reduction in patellofemoral loads. Hille [13] showed no effect on patellofemoral pressures or patellar contact surface area. Kelman and colleagues [7] showed that lateral release did not alter tracking or reduce pressure. Clinically, Unneberg and Reikerås [14] showed that 93% patients treated with lateral retinacular release failed to increase their activity level and only one (4%) returned to his preoperative sports level. Unneberg concluded that any "improvement in symptoms was more likely due to reduction in physical activity than the surgery." Osborne and Fulford [15] noted 87% good results at 1 year after lateral retinacular release but only 37% good results after 3 years. Christensen and colleagues [16] noted 24% poor results after lateral retinacular release at 1.2 years but 70% poor results at 4.6 years. Lindberg and colleagues [17] compared the results of physiotherapy with lateral retinacular release and found both groups to have 60% lack of improvement. This evidence does not support its routine use.

Patellar tracking

Van Kampen and Huiskes [18] noted that the three-dimensional motion of the patella consisted of flexion, wavering tilt, medial rotation, and lateral shift as the knee flexes, and that this tracking was controlled by the geometry of the trochlea and greatly influenced by the rotation of the tibia. He concluded that patellar tracking is highly susceptible to tibial rotations, which have a greater effect than either lateral retinacular release or tubercle elevation. He said that, to be valid, all biomechanical studies must take tibial rotation into consideration and that there was no experimental evidence to support the use of lateral retinacular release or anterior advancement of the tibial tubercle for the treatment of chondromalacia or the reduction of patellofemoral pressures. Kaatchburian

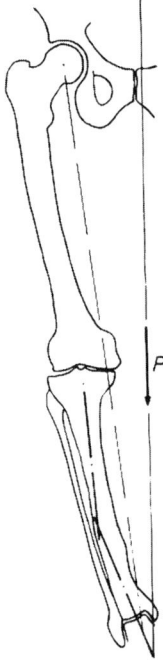

Fig. 10. Other conditions that shift the resultant vector medially include a varus fracture malunion, congenital varus of the femur or tibia, lateral ligament laxity, anterior cruciate ligament laxity, medial cartilage loss, or a medial transfer of the tibial tubercle. (*P*) Weight vector. (*From* Maquet PGJ. Biomechanics of the knee. Berlin: Springer-Verlag; 1976. p. 87; with permission.)

and colleagues [19] noted that accurate measurement of patellar tracking and even the definition of normal tracking have not yet been achieved in either experimental or clinical conditions. Therefore, there is little science to support using the diagnosis of patellar maltracking in surgical or other treatment decisions.

A framework for patient analysis: the basis for a better surgical strategy

A thorough literature review suggests that a new approach is needed to reduce and

---

Box 2. Failure mode of the four major anatomical structures

Skeleton: dysplasia
Cartilage: chondromalacia or arthrosis
Ligaments: instability
Muscle or tendon: tendinosus, weakness, or rupture

Box 3. To evaluate a PF joint

First: Look at the skeleton
Second: Look at the PF ligaments
Third: Look at the articular cartilage
Fourth: Look at the muscle/tendon unit

---

compartmentalize these multiple variables into some rational way. It would be helpful if there were a framework upon which to integrate and relate these many detailed observations. Searching a catalog of surgical techniques for the right solution is prone to lead to failure. On the contrary, the surgeon should "think biomechanics, think anatomy" and make this the basis of understanding pathomechanics. Such an analysis allows the clinician to devise the surgery that addresses the abnormal anatomy and thereby improves the biomechanics.

Biomechanics

The factors that increase patellofemoral articular pressure can be defined: (1) the total body weight, (2) the total muscle force needed to transmit the body weight to the ground, (3) the orientation of the skeleton beneath the muscle layer, (4) the length of the lever arms (height), and (5) the surface area that accepts the muscle force. Subluxation of the patella, for example, decreases the surface area for contact.

Paul Maquet's book *Biomechanics of the Knee* [20] is a masterly introduction to the concept of limb alignment. It covers concepts introduced by Pauwels and developed further by Maquet. However, it looks primarily at the coronal and sagittal planes with only a superficial consideration of the transverse plane. In Fig. 6, S_7 represents the center of gravity and the body mass that must be transmitted to the ground. The line of weight transference—vector P—falls medial to the knee joint. This creates a varus bending thrust. A valgus pull—vector L—created by the muscle (largely quadriceps) and the iliotibial track creates a second vector that, combined with vector P, gives us the resultant vector R, which acts on the center of the knee and is perpendicular to the tibial surface (Fig. 7). Fig. 8 shows the resultant vector R near the medial tibial spine and Fig. 9 shows that the consequence of increasing vector P or decreasing vector L is a medial shift of vector R with subsequent overload and wear of the medial compartment. Typically with

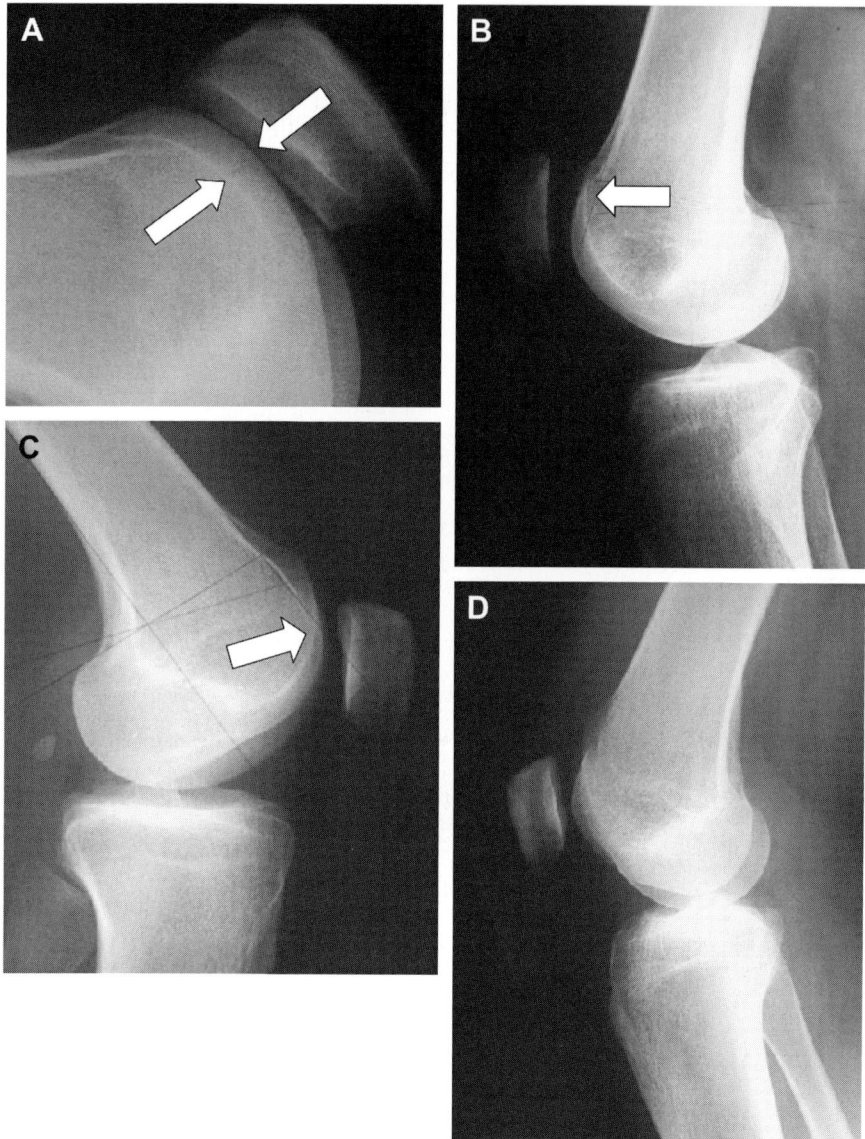

Fig. 11. (*A*) The trochlear depth (*area between arrows*) is seen on the true lateral radiograph in this normal knee. (*B*) Type 1 trochlear dysplasia. The depth of the trochlea becomes shallow (*arrow*) at the proximal articular surface as the trochlear floor crosses anterior to the anterior trochlear condyles. (*C*) Type 2 dysplasia. The floor of the trochlea crosses the condyles (*arrow*) well down the trochlea. (*D*) Type 3 dysplasia. The crossover occurs well down the trochlea and a CT scan will show a convex trochlea.

age, body weight (P) increases and muscle mass (L) decreases. Other causes of a medial shift of vector R include a varus fracture malunion, congenital varus of the femur or tibia, a laxity of the lateral collateral ligament, a laxity of the anterior cruciate ligament, a loss of medial compartment cartilage, or a medial transfer of the tibial tubercle (Fig. 10). The biomechanical consequence of medial tubercle transfer is medial compartment arthrosis (see Fig. 5) and medial facet arthritis (see Fig. 4).

Anatomy

This paradigm assumes that anatomy is normal because its design is the most optimal for function. Hence an abnormal anatomy does not

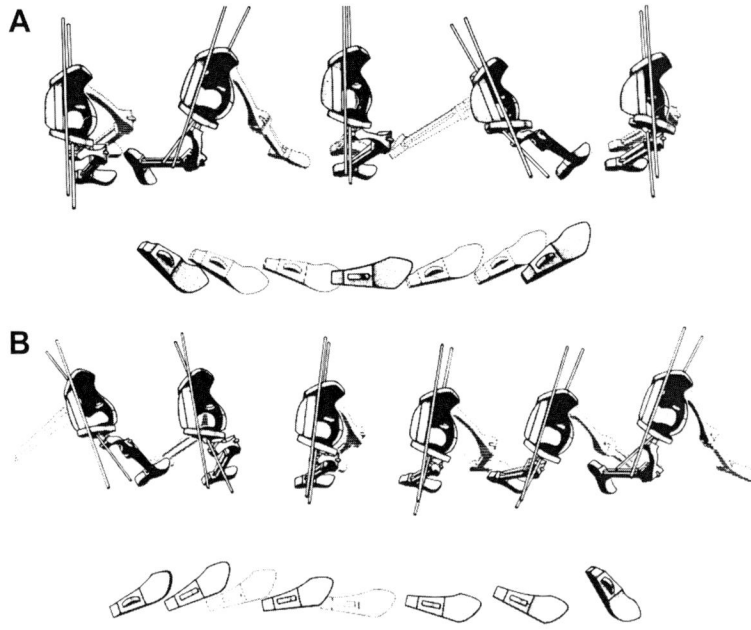

Fig. 12. The knee-joint axis normally rotates less than 10° internally and externally during gait. (*A*) Swinging leg is free to rotate internally from tow-off to heel strike. (*B*) Leg in stance phase and must rotate externally through the same amount. (*From* Saunders M, Inman VT, Eberhart HD. The major determinants in normal and pathological gait. In: Inham VT, Ralston HJ, Todd F. Human walking. Baltimore: Williams and Wilkins; 1981. p. 16; with permission.)

function as well. Anatomically there are only four major tissues to take into consideration: the skeleton, the muscles, the ligaments, and the cartilage. The skeleton creates the geometry that dictates the vector direction. Its length dictates how far the body mass is from the knee joint and the ground. The force provided by muscles and body weight dictate the magnitude of the vectors. Stability results from the ligaments acting against the skeleton. Cartilage reduces friction and transmits and distributes the force generated by the muscles. Pain may result from an abnormality of any or all of these four factors. It is critical when examining the patient to maintain an organized approach, remembering to assess each of these elements.

Other biological support systems, such as nerves, vessels, lymphatics, fat, and skin, can usually be ignored when examining for anterior knee pain, leaving only the four major anatomic tissues to consider and only four things that can go wrong (Box 2):

There may be an abnormal skeletal geometry or limb length or body mass that increases the load or, in the case of dysplasia, decreases intrinsic bony stability.

The articular cartilage may fail resulting in chondrosis or arthrosis.

The ligament may fail resulting in instability (subluxation or dislocation).

The tendon may fail (wear out) manifested as tendinopathy, attenuation, or rupture.

To evaluate the patient, independently assess each of these four structures. After the initial analysis try and relate these same structures to each other (Box 3).

Evaluate the skeleton

The skeleton is considered to have failed if it has an abnormal geometry. Brattström [21] showed in his series of patients with recurrent dislocation of the patella that a shallow sulcus was nearly always present. Dejour and colleagues [9] pointed out that this elevated shallow sulcus is best seen on a true lateral radiograph and he described three grades of dysplasia (Fig. 11A–D). The reshaping of the trochlear geometry requires bending or fracturing the subchondral plate, potentially damaging the articular cartilage. Because of this increased risk, reconstructing the failed ligament may be a safer but less direct approach.

Box 4. Factors to analyze in each anatomic plane

Coronal plane
　Varus-valgus
　Q-angle
　Pelvic width
　Mechanical axis limb inclination
　Patellar spin
　Heel valgus
Sagittal plane
　Recurvatum and knee flexion
　Patellar height Patellar flexion
　Tuberosity height
　Condylar radius of curvature
　Trochlear length
　Sulcus height
　Trochlear bump
Transverse plane
　Acetabular version
　Femoral torsion
　Tibial torsion
　Subtalar joint inclination
　Foot rotation
　Trochlear depth
　Tibial tuberosity–trochlear groove
　　distance

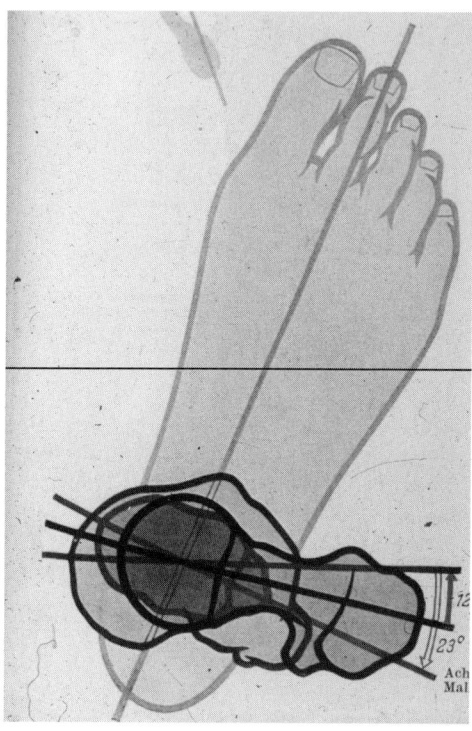

Fig. 13. Normal limb torsion in Lang is 12° femoral anteversion and 23° external tibial torsion. Yoskioka noted 13° femoral anteversion in both males and females but 21° external tibial torsion in males and 27° in females. (*From* Lang J, Wachsmuth W. Praktische anatomie, bein und static. Berlin: Springer-Verlag; 1972. p. 283; with permission.)

The abnormal geometry may also manifest itself as an abnormal skeletal axis. Skeletal malalignments include genu valgum or valgus, an abnormal femoral anteversion or retroversion, an abnormal recurvatum or flexion, an abnormal tibial torsion, and an abnormal hind foot or forefoot. Stan James' description of the patient with "miserable malalignment" is accurate, appropriate, and bears consideration in every patient with anterior knee pain [4]. It is the geometry of the skeleton that dictates where the body mass will be transmitted passing the knee joint to the ground. A skeleton out of normal alignment may cause an abnormally high displacement force to be exerted on the patella. This force is commonly due to the knee joint twisting out of the plane of forward body motion and is usually due to a skeletal malalignment. This skeletal malalignment is, however, not the same as patellar malalignment frequently cited in patellofemoral literature. Too much of a displacement force may be created by an "inward pointing knee," which may be due to an abnormal increase in femoral anteversion, an abnormal increase in external tibial torsion, an abnormal hyperpronation of the foot, a contracture of the Achilles tendon, genu valgum, or a weakness of hip external rotators. The position of the knee joint moving in space between the center of mass and the ground, the speed of this motion, the length of the lever arms, and the mass combine to determine the forces on the patellofemoral joint. Normally the knee-joint axis moves internally relative to the pelvis during the stance phase and externally relative to the pelvis during the swing phase of gait (Fig. 12). If the knee-joint axis is pointed medially while the body is moving forward, there is an excess lateral pull on the patella, which increases stress on the medial retinaculum and medial patellofemoral ligaments, reduces weight-bearing on the medial patellofemoral articular cartilage, and creates excess compression on the lateral facet and lateral trochlea. If the excess stress on the medial ligament is sufficient, the ligament may fail,

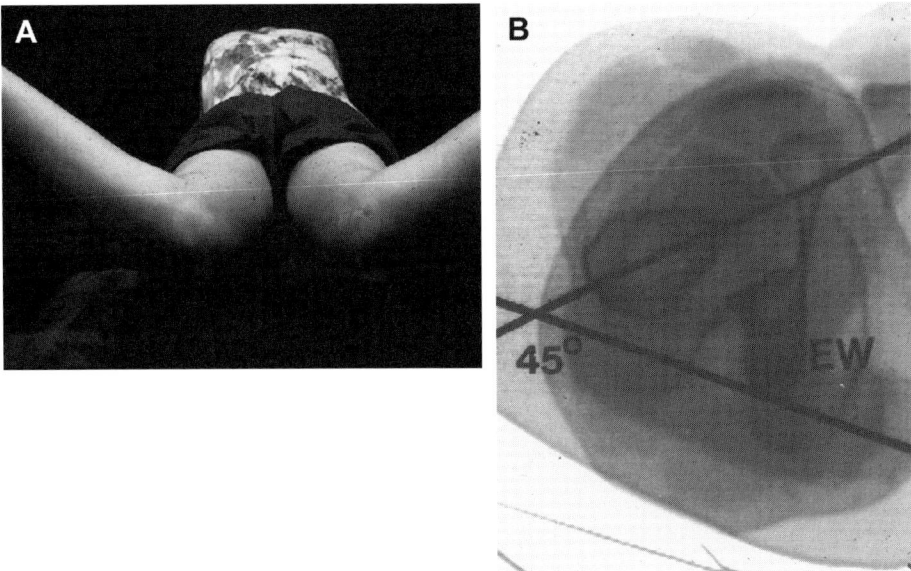

Fig. 14. (*A*) Internal rotation of the hip is measured in extension. This 18-year-old female had femoral anteversion of 45°. At age 12, she developed anterior knee pain, and at age 15 she dislocated the patella playing hockey. After medial patellofemoral ligament reconstruction, she had recurrent pain with the patella giving way. After 30° rotational osteotomy of femur, she returned to sports without restriction or symptoms. (*B*) CT scan of patient with anterior knee pain and eventual dislocation patella. Patient was symptomatic after medial patellofemoral ligament reconstruction but asymptomatic after 30° external rotation osteotomy.

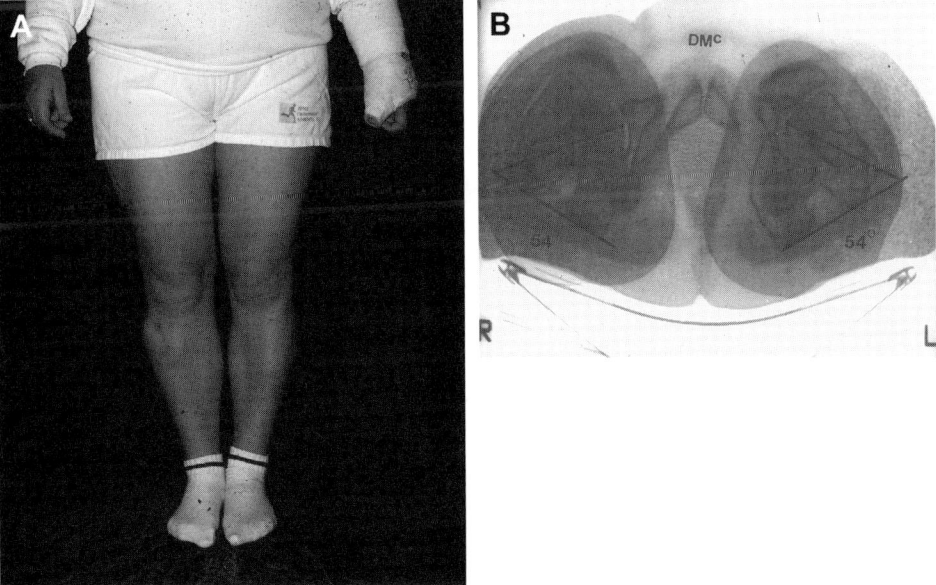

Fig. 15. Abnormal femoral torsion is not always obvious. (*A*) Patient with multiple failed surgeries, including a failed Maquet osteotomy with skin breakdown and gastroc nemius flap on the right. Patient is shown here 3 months post–40° intertrochanteric rotational osteotomy of the right femur. (*B*) CT rotational study of above patient showing a femoral anteversion of 54°. At 8 weeks post–40° external rotation osteotomy, she wanted the other side done because she could already feel less stress in the right knee.

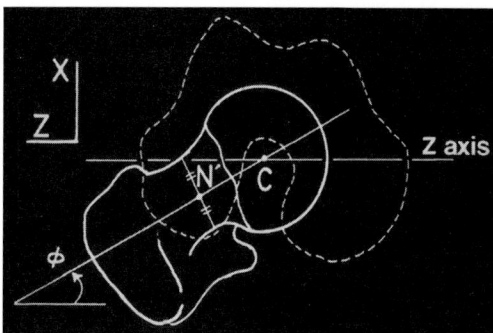

Fig. 16. The method of Murphy uses a line between the center of the femoral head and the center of the femoral neck against a line tangent to the posterior surface of the femoral condyles or between the epicondyles. The Z axis passes through the femoral epicondyles. C, center of the femoral head; N, width of the neck of the femur; X, x axis; Z, z axis; ø, angle of anteversion of the femur. (*From* Yoshioka Y, Siu D, Cooke TD. The anatomy and functional axes of the femur. J Bone Joint Surg Am 1987;69:875; with permission.)

resulting in lateral subluxation or dislocation and a secondary reduction in contact surface area. If the ligament does not fail, the excess force may result in gradual destruction of the lateral patellofemoral articular cartilage. Alternative skeletal malalignments result in analogous biomechanical overloads. There is no imaging technique that measures in situ forces.

The limb skeleton must be analyzed in all three planes (Box 4).

Skeletal alignment in the horizontal plane is not usually evaluated. However, James [22], Takai and colleagues [23], Janssen [24], Laret and colleagues [25], Stroud and colleagues [26], Winson and colleagues [27], Delgado and colleagues [28], Eckhoff and colleagues [29], Powers [30], Lee and colleagues [31], and others have made correlations between abnormal limb torsion and patellofemoral pain, instability, or arthritis. Normal torsional alignment measurements are usually in the range shown in Fig. 13 by Lang and Wachsmuth [32]. Yoshioka and colleagues [33,34] reviewed the literature on femoral anteversion and suggested an osteology measurement standard and an average of 13° of femoral anteversion was present in the specimens he studied.

The physical examination for skeletal torsion is best done with the subject prone because this position is closer to the hip position during gait. Internal (Fig. 14A, B) and external hip rotation

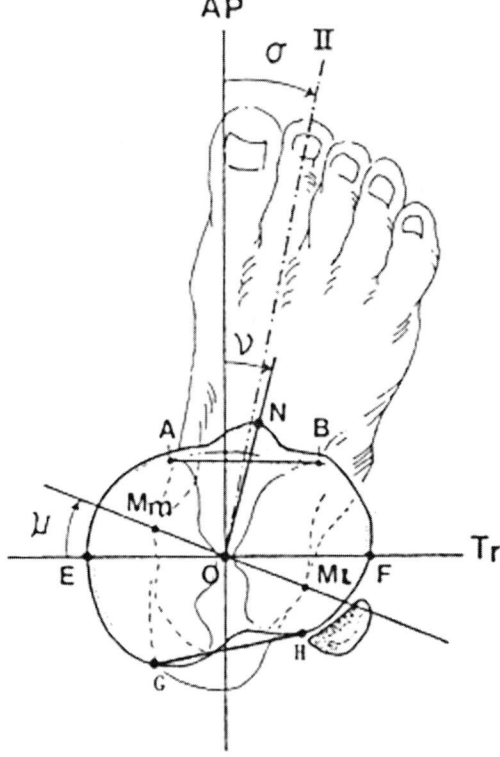

Fig. 17. Tibial torsion (μ) measured across the transverse axis of the plateau (Tr) and the malleoli (Mm–ML). σ, measure of foot outward rotation; II, axis of the second ray; ν, lateral deviation of the tibial tuberosity; A, anterior margin of the medial articular surface of the tibial plateau; AP, anterior-posterior axis of the tibial plateau and represents the X axis; B, anterior margin of the lateral articular surface of the tibial plateau; E, most medial border of the tibial plateau as measured along the transverse axis Tr; F, most lateral border of the tibial plateau as measured on the transverse axis Tr; G, posterior margin of the articular surface of the medial tibial plateau articular surface; H, the most posterior margin of the lateral tibial plateau articular margin; ML, center of the lateral malleolus; MM, center of the medial malleolus; N, peak of the tibial tuberosity; O, knee center. (*From* Yoshioka Y, Siu D, Cooke TD, et al. Tibial anatomy and functional axes. J Orthop Res 1989:7(1);133; reprinted with permission of Wiley-Liss, Inc., a subsidiary of John Wiley & Sons, Inc.)

give an indication of femoral torsion and the foot-thigh axis may give an indication of tibial torsion. The clinical findings may be easily missed as seen in Fig. 15A. The CT scan (Fig. 15B) is used for the definitive measurement using the method of Murphy and colleagues [35] (Fig. 16) for the femur and abstracting from Yoshioka and colleagues [36] for the tibial torsion (Fig. 17).

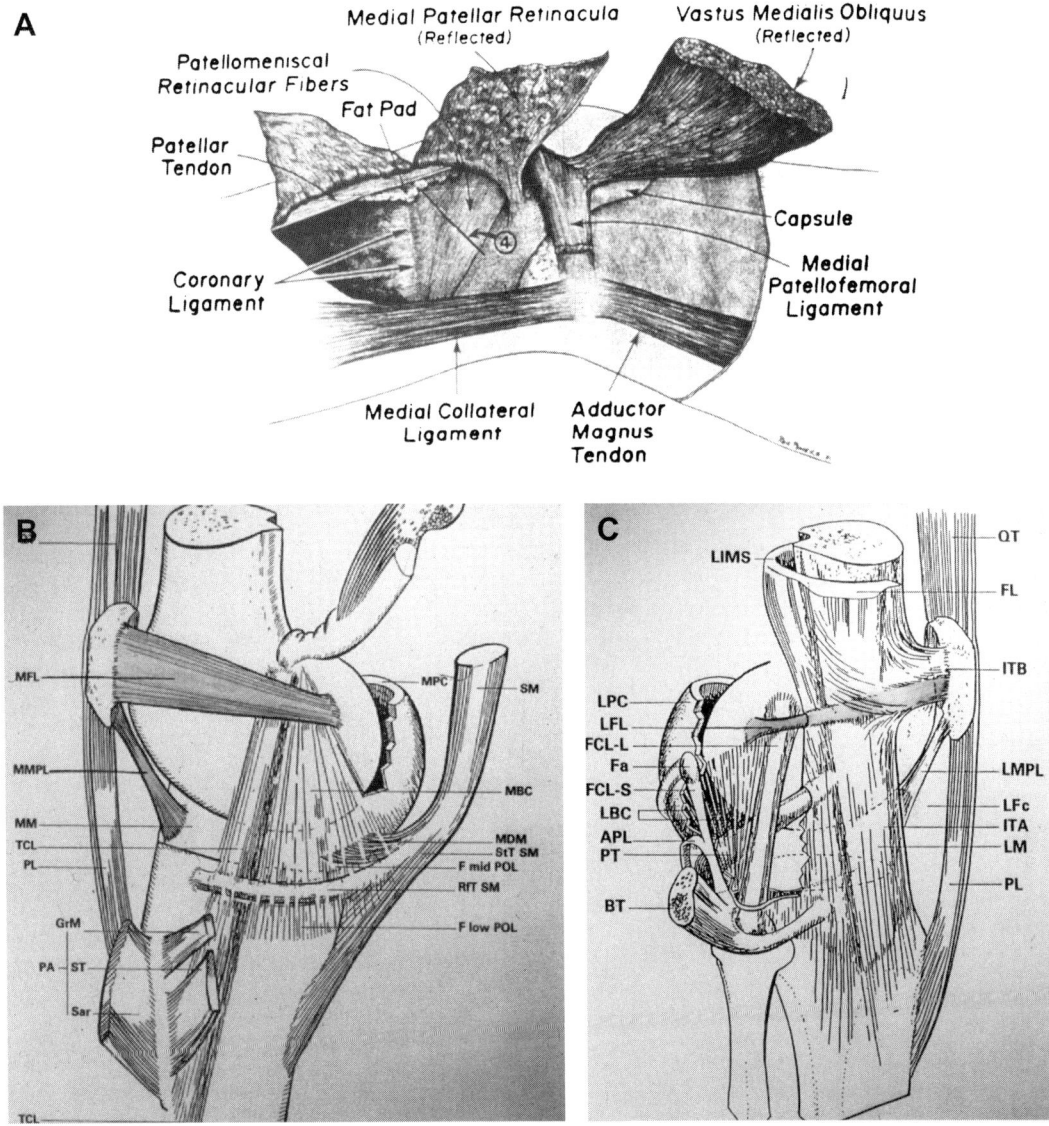

Fig. 18. (*A*) Medial patellofemoral ligament as depicted by Conlon. (4) Line of sectioning of the medial meniscopatellar ligament. (*B*) Depictions of the medial patellofemoral ligament and the meniscopatellar ligament. F low POL, lower fascicles Posterior Oblique Ligament; F mid POL, me\id portion posterior oblique ligament; GrM, gracilis muscle; MFL, Medial Patellofemoral Ligament; MM, medial meniscus; MMPL, medial meniscopatellar ligament; MPC, meial posterior capsule; PA, pes Anserinus; PL, patellar ligament; QT, Quadriceps tendon; RfT SM, reflected tendon semimembranosus; Sar, sartorius; SM, semimembranosus; ST, semitendinosus; StT SM, straight tendon semimembranosus; TCL, tibial collateral ligament. (*C*) The lateral patellofemoral ligament, lateral meniscopatellar ligament, and anterior sweeping fibers of the iliotibial band all contribute to preventing medial patellar subluxation, but also add to the resistance preventing lateral patella displacement. APL, Arcuate-popliteal ligament; BT, biceps tendon; Fa, fabella; FCL-L, fibular collateral ligament -long; FCL-S, fibular collateral ligament-short; FL, fascia lata; ITA, Iliotibial attachment; ITB, iliotibial band; Lfc, lateral fat pad; LFL, lateral patellofemoral ligament; LIMS, lateral intermuscular septum; LM, lateral meniscus; LMPL, lateral meniscopatellar ligament; LPC, lateral posterior capsule; PL, patellar ligament; PT, popliteal tendon; QT, quadriceps tendon. (*From* Conlan T, Garth Jr. WP, Lemons JE. Evaluation of the medial soft tissue restraints of the extensor mechanism of the knee. J Bone Joint Surg Am 1993:75;686; with permission.)

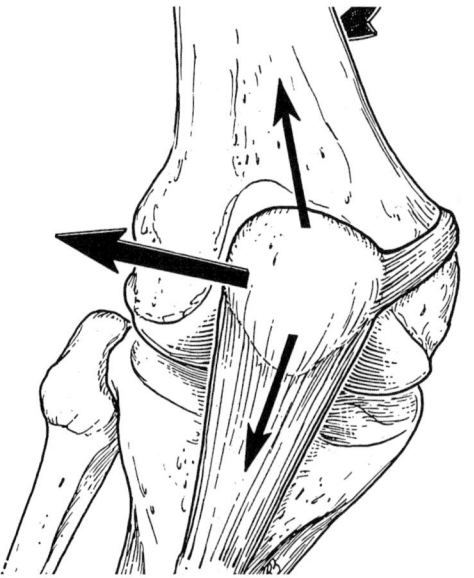

Fig. 19. The quadriceps pull on the patella is normally lateral and is normally balanced by the trochlear depth and the medial patellofemoral ligament. (*Large arrow* denotes the lateral displacement vector pulling on the patella created by the vertical *upward arrow* representing the quadriceps vector and the *downward arrow* representing the patellar tendon. This lateral pull is increased with an inward twist of the femur or an outward twist of the tibia and is resisted by the medial patellofemoral ligament shown connecting the medial epicondylar region of the femur with the superior medial border of the patella.) (*From* Teitge RA. Treatment of complications of patellofemoral joint surgery. In: Operative techniques in sports medicine. Philadelphia: WB Saunders; 1994. p. 331; with permission.)

Evaluate patellofemoral ligaments

The primary stabilizer of the patellofemoral joint preventing lateral dislocation is the medial patellofemoral ligament as Conlon [37] first demonstrated biomechanically that the MPFL was the primary stabilizer (Fig. 18A, B). There are three stabilizers resisting lateral patellar displacement. These are most importantly the medial retinacular ligaments, next in importance the trochlear geometry and lastly the lateral retinaculum. The medial patellofemoral ligament part of the medial retinaculum affords the most resistance while the meniscopatellar ligament is the second most important restraint. The secondary stabilizer is the trochlear geometry and third is the lateral retinaculum (see Fig. 18C). The ligaments and trochlear groove resist the normal lateral pull of the quadriceps (Fig. 19). The dynamic evaluation of any ligament function requires the application of a force and the measurement of the resulting displacement. To evaluate patellofemoral ligaments, the author prefers stress radiography (Fig. 20A, B) [38].

The patella must be stressed in both the medial and the lateral directions as it can dislocate or subluxate in either direction. Stress radiography is used routinely before every patellar instability surgery. Fig. 21A shows the patellofemoral joint radiograph in a patient with a knee that buckles without warning. The radiographic parameters are completely normal. Stress radiography (Fig. 21B) shows the patella dislocated completely in the lateral direction. Without stress radiography, the diagnosis could easily be missed. For

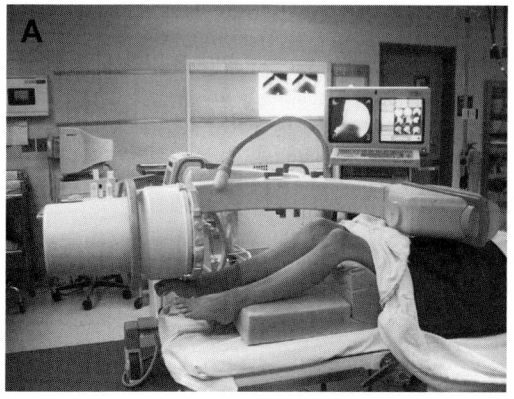
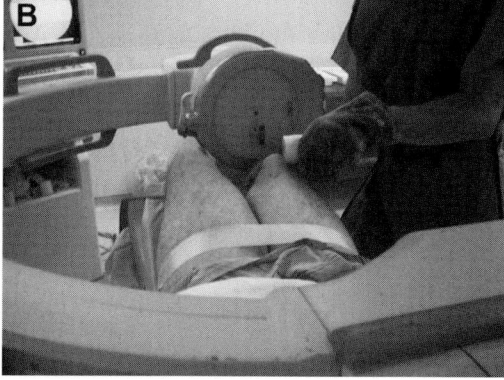

Fig. 20. (*A*) Intraoperative setup for documentation of patellar laxity using stress radiographs and the image intensifier. (*B*) Application of stress for documenting medial patellar laxity.

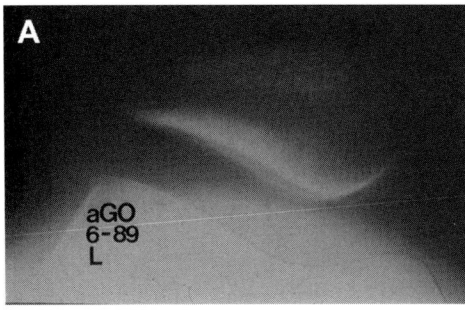
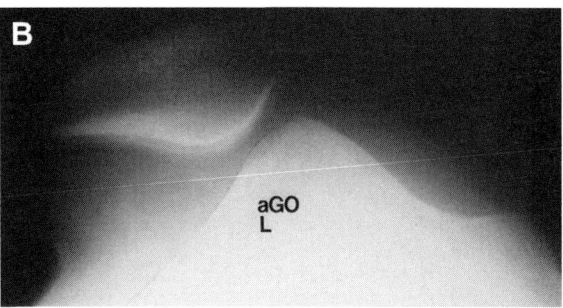

Fig. 21. (A) Axial patellofemoral radiograph of patient with anterior knee pain and appreciation with lateral patellar stress. Plain radiographic parameters used to diagnose patellar instability are all normal. (B) When a lateral stress is applied to the patella, it readily dislocated. This case emphasizes the need for a stress examination and documentation when searching for instability.

a lateral dislocation to occur, the medial patellofemoral ligaments must have failed.

Lateral retinacular release often results in further loss of lateral stability and allows the patella to be displaced excessively in the medial direction. At the 1990 American Academy of Orthopaedic Surgeons meeting, a series of 70 patients subjectively worse after lateral release were shown to have medial patellar dislocation when stress radiography was used for diagnosis (Fig. 22A, B).

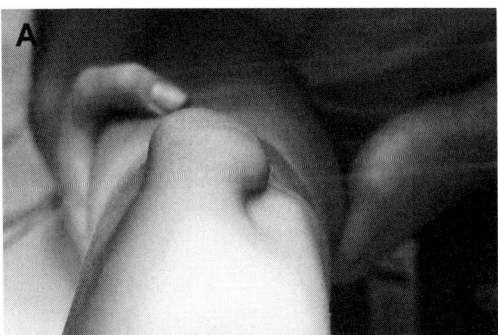
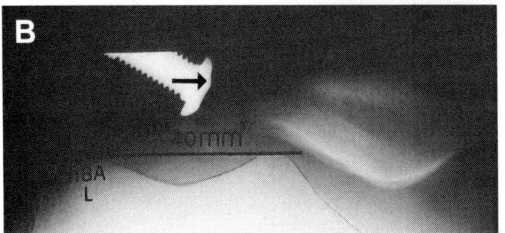

Fig. 22. (A) A medial dislocated patella after prior lateral retinacular release. (B) Stress radiograph of a patella for diagnosis of medial dislocation.

Evaluate articular cartilage

To evaluate articular cartilage, the author prefers the double-contrast CT-arthrogram. Ultimately, of course, MRI will supplant it, but to date, at Michigan Orthopaedic Specialty Hospital, the resolution has been better with CT than with magnetic resonance (Fig. 23A–D). Some lesions of course are seen better with arthroscopy, but there is difficulty determining a precise location of the lesion, the surface area measurement, and especially the depth on the lesion when subchondral bone is not exposed. The depth of the lesion is generally well seen on the CT-arthrogram.

Evaluate the muscle and tendon

The understanding of the pathophysiology of tendonopathy remains unknown What is recognized is the lack of an inflammatory response in the diseased tendon. It has been stated that all successful treatments have as a common denominator the stimulation of an inflammatory response necessary for healing. Kannus and Jozsa [39], in a review of the pathology of ruptured tendons, found anoxic mitochondria to be the common feature in all. Quadriceps muscle atrophy may be quite severe in cases of patellar or quadriceps tendinosus and this atrophy is presumed to be due to disuse secondary to chronic pain.

Summary for evaluation of the patellofemoral joint

As stated in Box 3, an evaluation of the patellofemoral joint begins with a look at the skeleton, then the ligaments, then the articular cartilage, and finally the muscle and tendon.

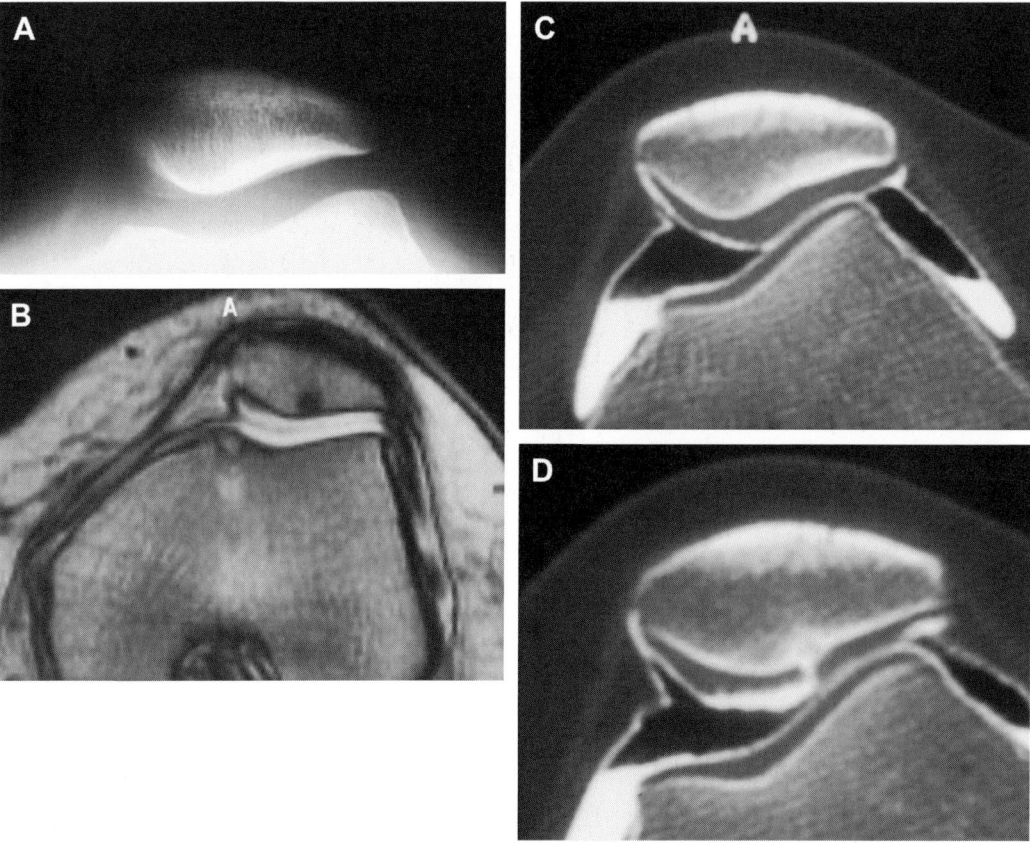

Fig. 23. (*A*) Axial view of patellofemoral joint in 23-year-old student with retropatellar pain after minor twisting injury. (*B*) MRI showing lesion in subchondral bone. Radiologist called this avascular necrosis. Two orthopaedic surgeons recommended biopsy (A). (*C*) Double-contrast CT-arthrogram at level just above the lesion. Note lateral subluxation, increased subchondral sclerosis in the lateral facet, and indentation of the patellar articular cartilage caused by the lateral patellar position (A). (*D*) Double-contrast CT-arthrogram at the level of the lesion. Note the compression of articular cartilage lateral to the lesion, but a vertical split in the articular cartilage extending down to the subchondral bone where a cyst has developed, and the inspisation of dye into the articular cartilage medial to the split cartilage. This is the pattern seen with a lateral dislocation where the patella moved up the lateral trochlear wall until the cartilage failed, causing the vertical split and, with further lateral displacement, the lamina splendens is scraped off the medial ridge of the patella. The treatment recommended was a medial patellofemoral ligament reconstruction.

Changing the skeleton changes the ligament stress and the cartilage loading. Addressing the ligaments or the cartilage does not change the skeleton. If the knee joint is moving sideways (pointing inward) (Fig. 24) while the body is moving forward, a shear force is created, straining the medial retinaculum and compressing the lateral facet (Fig. 25).

The message regarding patellofemoral biomechanics is that sometimes you cannot pull the patella back onto the femur. You must rotate the femur back underneath the patella (Fig. 26). The patellofemoral joint must be looked at not as only the patella and trochlear but as the orientation of the knee joint relative to the torso above and the foot and ground below.

In summary, the skeleton determines where in space the patellofemoral joint is placed between the body's center of mass and the ground. Changes in skeletal geometry change where the body weight crosses the knee joint as it is transferred to the ground. The alignment factors that change the direction of force transmission include tibial torsion, genu varum or valgum, femoral torsion, pronated feet, subtalar inclination, plantar flexed first ray, and tight Achilles. The

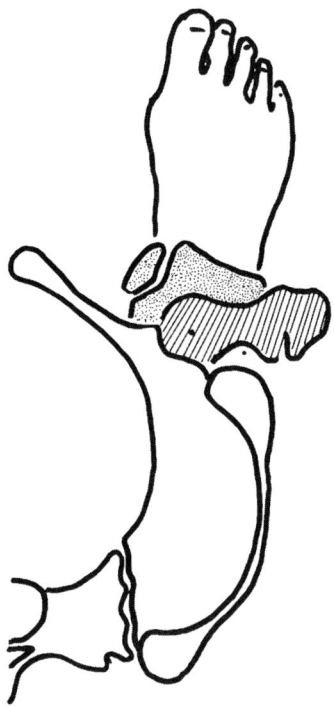

Fig. 24. If the knee joint is moving sideways while the body is moving forward, then the patella moves laterally, stressing the medial stabilizing ligaments and increasing compression on the lateral facet while decreasing compression on the medial facet. (Oblique lines indicate the proximal femur [head, neck, and greater trochanter]; shaded area indicates the distal femur and patella.)

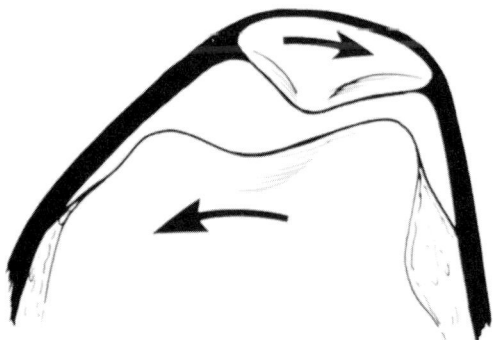

Fig. 25. If the femur rotates internally, it twists (*lower arrow*) out from underneath the patella, which is then moving laterally (*upper arrow*) pulling on the medial retinaculum and compressing the lateral facet. (*From* Teitge RA. Treatment of complications of patellofemoral joint surgery. In: Operative techniques in sports medicine. Philadelphia: WB Saunders; 1994. p. 322; with permission.)

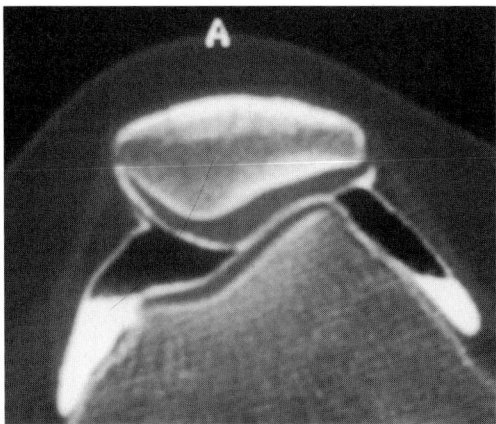

Fig. 26. If this lateral patellar subluxation is due to limb torsional malalignment, you can't pull the patella back onto the trochlea. You must rotate the limb back under the patella (A).

components in the knee that accept the vector of body weight transmission are the patellofemoral ligaments, the articular cartilage and underlying bone, and the quadriceps and patellar tendons.

Surgical strategy: putting it all together

The goal of operative treatment is to normalize the biomechanics through restitution of normal anatomy. The morbidity of surgery may dictate otherwise. When multiple anatomic abnormalities are present, it is not known which may be more important. If a patient has patellofemoral cartilage damage, recurrent lateral patellar subluxation, trochlear dysplasia, a femoral anteversion of 45°, an external tibial torsion of 45°, a genu valgum of 10°, a patella alta, and a contracture of the Achilles, is it best to perform a varus, external rotation femoral osteotomy, with an internal rotation tibial osteotomy; a trochlear osteotomy; a medial patellofemoral ligament reconstruction; a distalization of the tibial tubercle; and an Achilles lengthening? These abnormal anatomic findings are often subtle but combinations of pathologies are quite common. This surgical approach of correcting all abnormalities is quite logical from the biomechanical standpoint, but excessive from the surgical morbidity standpoint. A biomechanical solution may mean that the ligament reconstruction is not necessary because the displacing forces are reduced, and a cartilage restoration is not necessary because the compression forces are reduced and changed in

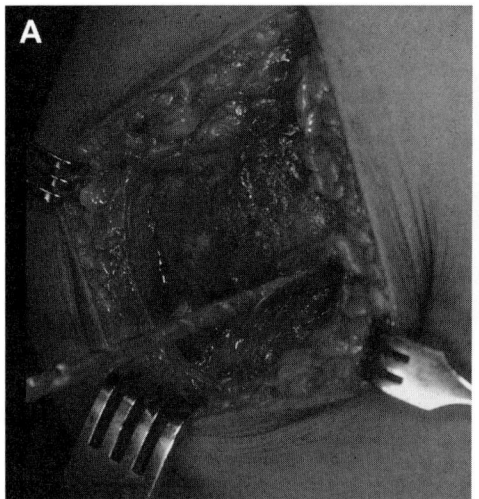
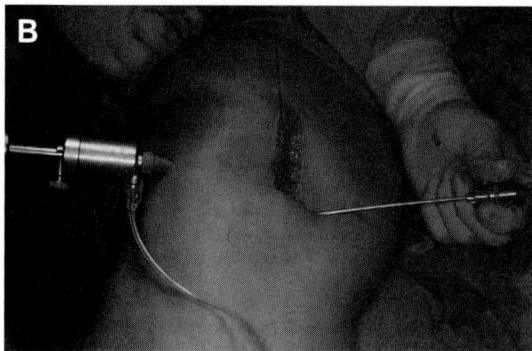

Fig. 27. (*A*) An adductor tendon graft is left attached to the adductor tubercle and tunneled through the medial femoral condyle to the isometric point, then passed deep to the vastus medialis to be inserted into the superior medial patella deep to the upper left retractor. (*B*) The isometric point near the medial epicondyle is located with a Kirschner wire moved around the epicondylar region. A string is run from this point to an isometer, which is inserted into the lateral patella. The change in distance between the Kirschner wire and the superior medial patella is measured while the knee is flexed and extended.

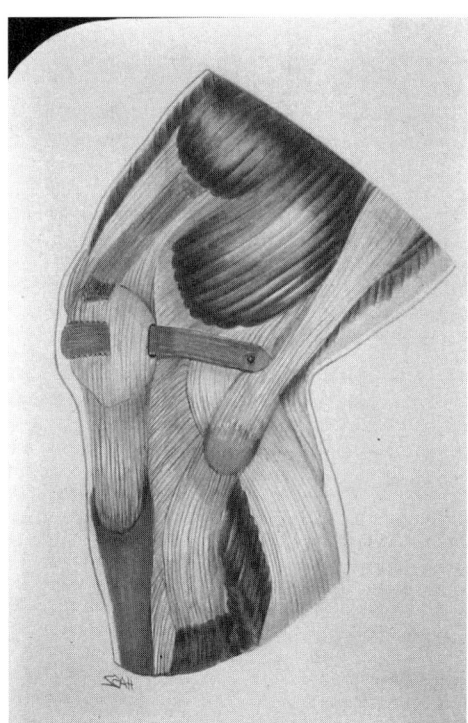

Fig. 28. A lateral patellofemoral ligament reconstruction has been used since 1981 for treatment of iatrogenic medial dislocation. Here a quadriceps tendon was used for the graft. (*Courtesy of* Heide Siklich-Zerilli.)

location. As yet, no biomechanical studies indicate which surgery alters biomechanics the most.

If the skeletal alignment is normal and instability exists because of ligament injury or ligament injury exists with a shallow trochlea, ligament reconstruction may be appropriate. The author has used a reconstruction of the medial patellofemoral ligament for over 20 years as the primary treatment of lateral instability. The choice of graft material is optional, but the location in which it is put must reconstruct the normal tension behavior. An isometric graft is not likely to overcompress the patellofemoral articular cartilage during knee flexion (Fig. 27A, B). If stress radiographs indicate a medial patella dislocation, then a lateral patellofemoral ligament reconstruction developed in 1981 is used (Fig. 28).

If the skeletal alignment is normal, the ligaments are normal, and there is severe cartilage loss, fresh allograft replacement may be considered. A follow-up at an average of 10 years postreplacement of both trochlea and patella yielded some exceptional results (Figs. 29 and 30A, B).

The surgical strategy is summarized in Box 5. Fig. 31 summarizes the relationship of causes of anterior knee pain. Fig. 32 summarizes treatments related to surgical strategy.

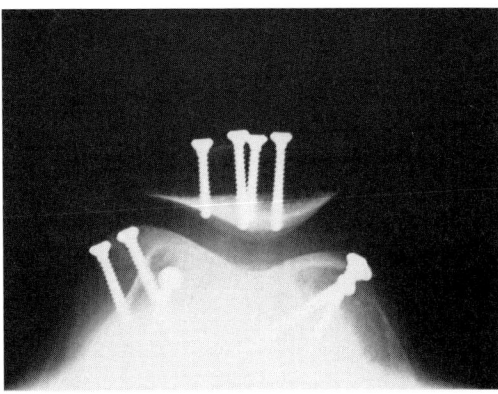

Fig. 29. A fresh bipolar allograft may be a salvage for patellofemoral arthrosis.

Case study analysis

Case 1: (see Figs. 1 and 2) A 42-year-old law-enforcement officer presented 20 years after he dislocated patella playing college football, and was treated with a medial tibial tubercle transfer and lateral retinacular release (Fig. 33A–C). He

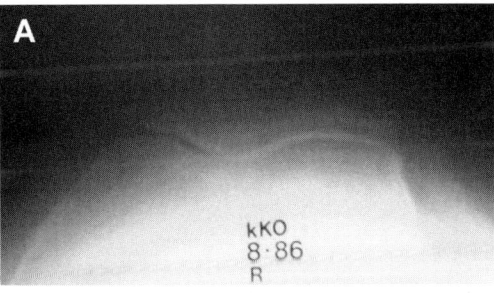

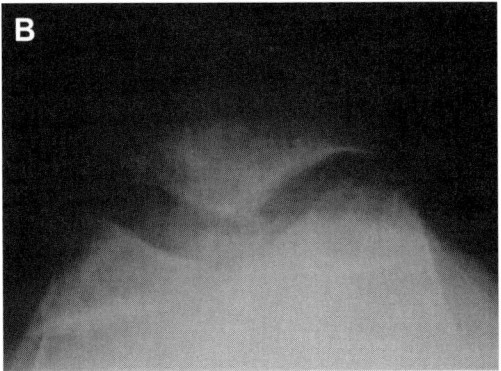

Fig. 30. (*A*) Axial patellar radiograph of 32-year-old woman with patellofemoral arthrosis. (*B*) Axial view of same patient 16 years after fresh bipolar osteochondral shell allograft.

Box 5. Summary of surgical treatments

Skeletal malalignment treatments
For excess femoral anteversion, do external rotation femoral osteotomy
For decreased femoral anteversion, do internal rotation femoral osteotomy
For excess external tibial torsion, do internal rotation tibial osteotomy
For decreased tibial torsion, do external rotation tibial osteotomy
For trochlear dysplasia, do trochlear osteotomy

Instability treatments
For ligament insufficiency, do ligament reconstruction
For trochlear insufficiency, do trochlear osteotomy

Arthrosis (cartilage loss) treatments
Rebalance the patellofemoral load with limb osteotomy
Recenter the patella with ligament reconstruction
Replace the cartilage with:
 Fresh allograft
 Prosthesis
 Other future technologies

has pain with all walking and riding in a car. Before considering a prosthesis, evaluate the skeletal alignment. The ligaments and cartilage condition is obviously poor (Fig. 33D). Coronal alignment (full standing lower limb) shows 5° genu valgum. Horizontal alignment (Fig. 33E, F) shows 38° femoral anteversion, 19° external tibial torsion. The initial treatment was a 5° varus and 25° external rotation distal femoral osteotomy with a medial patellofemoral ligament reconstruction (Fig. 33G, H). He was able to return to light exercise and painless walking (Fig. 33I, J).

Case 2: (see Fig. 3) Before considering microfracture, osteoarticular transfer system, Maquet/Bandi, Fulkerson/Beckers, lateral release, or prosthesis in this 28-year-old athlete in too much pain to continue to play softball or volleyball, break the problem into its components. First, look at the skeleton in the coronal, sagittal, and horizontal planes. The condition of the ligaments and articular cartilage is obvious on

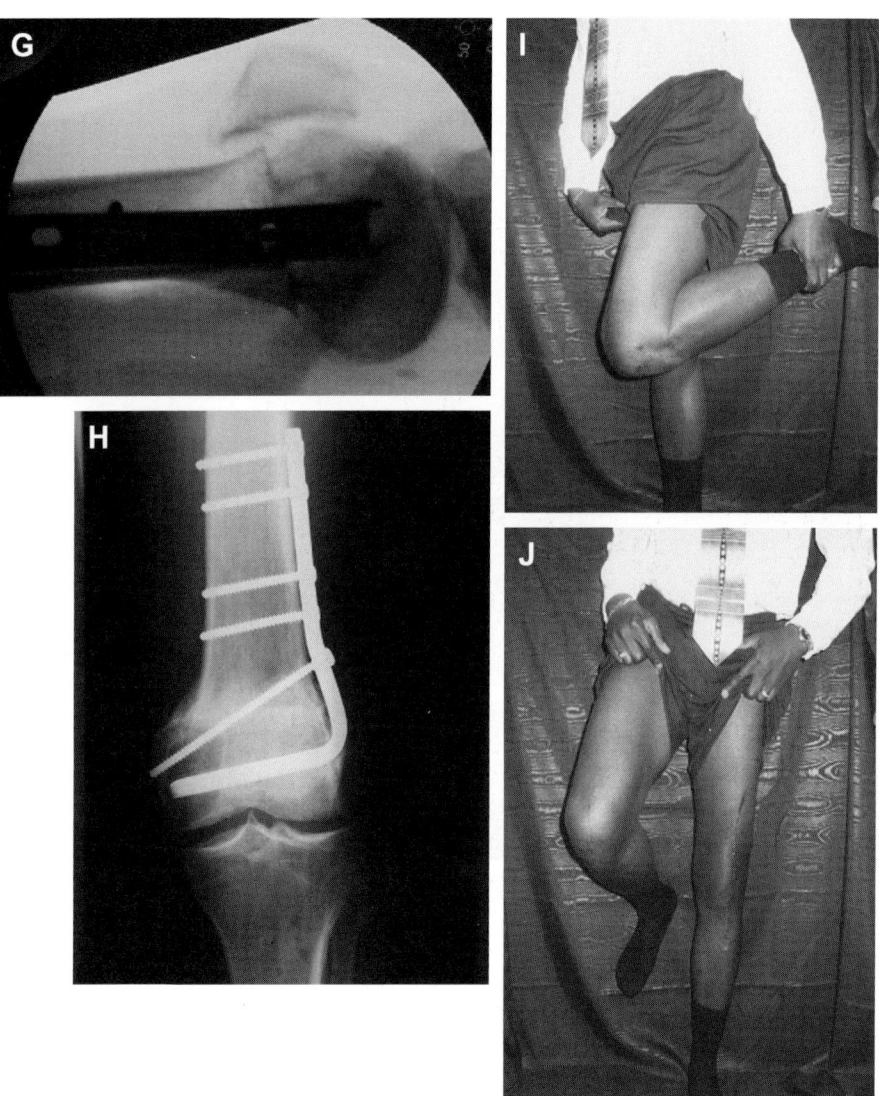

Fig. 33 (*continued*).

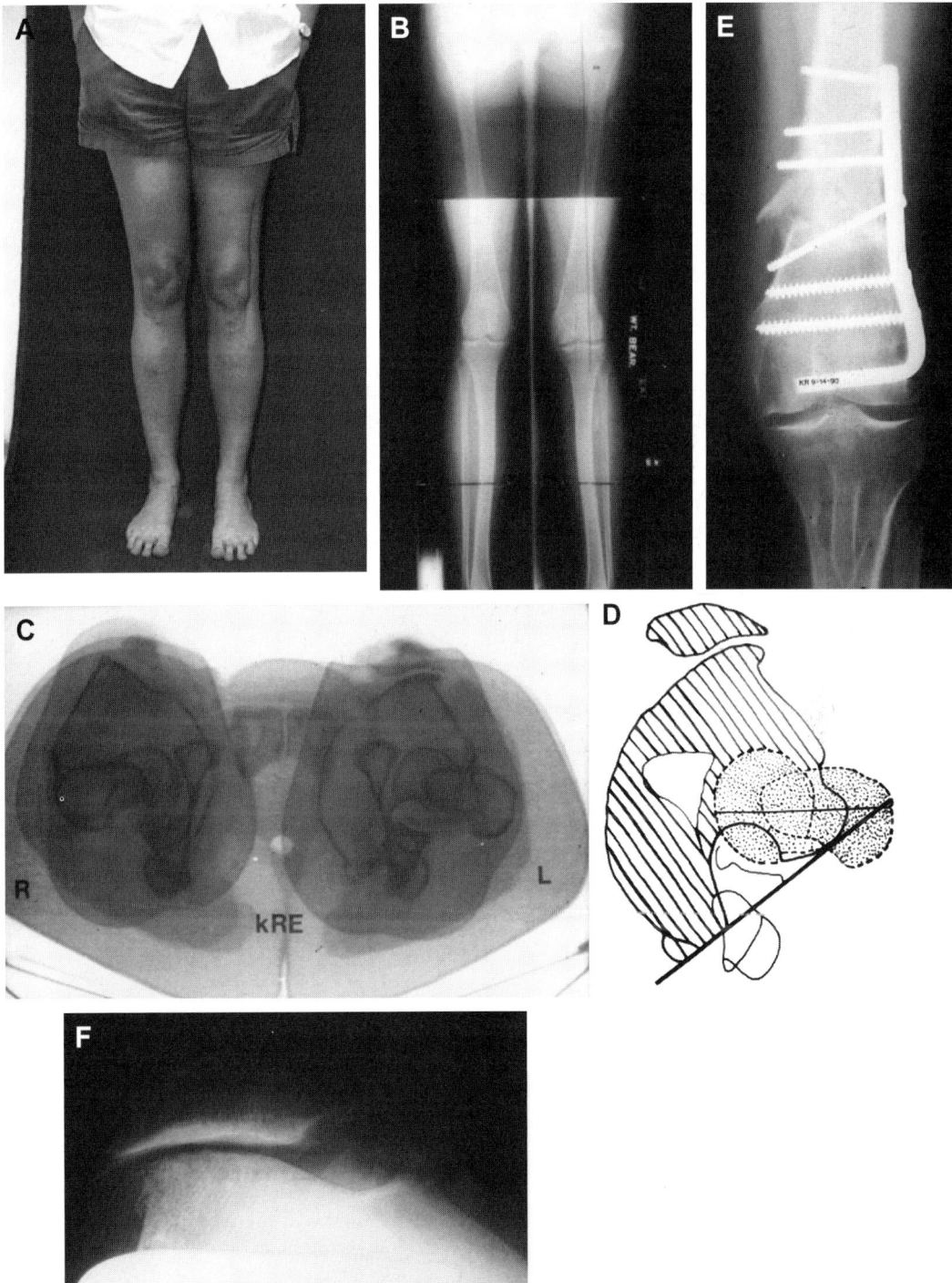

Fig. 34. (A) Mild genu valgum seen on the right. The left is postosteotomy. (B) The whole limb standing radiograph shows mechanical axis in the lateral compartment. (C) CT rotational study confirms increase in femoral anteversion. (D) Preoperative tracing of femoral anteversion measures 35°. (E) Radiograph post–20° external rotation, 5° varus osteotomy with distalization of the tubercle for patella alta. (F) Radiograph 4.5 years postosteotomy showing the development of a joint space. She had returned to playing softball. Contrast this with Fig. 3.

the axial patellofemoral radiograph (see Fig. 3). Fig. 34A shows a limb to be in valgus. The whole leg standing radiograph (Fig. 34B) confirms and quantifies the valgus. Fig. 34C and D show the horizontal plane to have an excess of femoral anteversion. A sagittal radiograph confirmed patella alta. Physical examination shows long limbs (see Fig. 34A). For treatments, first put the femur back under the patella. This was accomplished with a 5° varus, 22° external rotation distal femoral osteotomy and distalization transfer of the tibial tubercle. Fig. 34F shows the axial patellofemoral radiograph at a 4-year follow-up. She had returned to both softball and volleyball.

Summary

This article made five main points:

Bone architecture dictates where the force vectors acting on the patella will be directed.

Abnormal skeletal alignment may alter the displacement forces acting on the patellofemoral joint, causing ligament failure with subsequent instability.

Skeletal malalignment may also increase patellar facet loading leading to arthrosis.

Increased joint loading with the addition of subluxation may further increase unit loading. Pain results from this excess load and tension in the soft tissue or compression of articular surfaces.

Treatment depends on the primary pathology. With a large displacement force and failed ligaments, the best treatment may be both osteotomy of long bones and ligament reconstruction.

References

[1] Tomsich DA, Nitz AJ, Threlkeld AJ, et al. Patellofemoral alignment: reliability. J Orthop Sports Phys Ther 1996;23:200–8.

[2] Greene CG, Edwards TB, Wade MR, et al. Reliability of the quadriceps angle measurement. Am J Knee Surg 2001;14:97–103.

[3] Insall J, Falvo KA, Wise DW. Chondromalacia patellae, a prospective study. J Bone Joint Surg Am 1976;58:1–8.

[4] Kuroda R, Kambic H, Valdevit A, et al. Articular cartilage contact pressures after tibial tubercle transfer—a cadaveric study. Am J Sports Med 2001;29:403–9.

[5] Ostermeier S, Stukenborg-Colsman C, Hurschler C, et al. In vitro investigation of the effect of medial patellofemoral ligament reconstruction and medial tibial tuberosity transfer on lateral patellar stability. Arthroscopy 2006;22:308–19.

[6] Huberti HH, Hayes WC. Patellofemoral contact pressures. The influence of q-angle and tendofemoral contact. J Bone Joint Surg Am 1984;66:715–24.

[7] Kelman GJ, Focht L, Drakauer JD, et al. A cadaveric study of patellofemoral kinematics using a biomechanical testing rig and gait laboratory motion analysis. Orthopaedic Transactions 1989;13:248–9.

[8] Huber J, Gasser B, Perren SM, et al. Changes in retropatellar pressure values in relation to the position of the tibial tuberosity. Knee 1994;1(Suppl 1):19–43.

[9] Dejour H, Walch G, Nove-Josserand L, et al. Factors of patellar instability: an anatomic radiographic study. Knee Surg Sports Traumatol Arthrosc 1994;2:19–26.

[10] Hughston J, Walsh WM. Proximal and distal reconstruction of the extensor mechanism for patellar subluxation. Clin Orthop Relat Res 1979;144:40.

[11] Christoforakis J, Bull AMJ, Strachan RK, et al. Effects of lateral retinacular release on the lateral stability of the patella. Knee Surg Sports Traumatol Arthrosc 2006;14:273–7.

[12] Huberti HH, Hayes WC. Contact pressures in chondromalacia patellae and the effects of capsular reconstructive procedures. J Orthop Res 1988;6:499–508.

[13] Hille E. Pressure and contact-surface measurements within the femoropatellar joint and their variations following lateral release. Archives of Orthopaedic and Traumatic Surgery 1988;107:226–7.

[14] Unneberg K, Reikerås O. The effect of lateral retinacular release in idiopathic chondromalacia patellae. Arch Orthop Trauma Surg 1988;107:226–7.

[15] Osborne AH, Fulford PC. Lateral release for chondromalacia patallae. J Bone Joint Surg Br 1982;64:202–5.

[16] Christensen F, Søballe K, Snerum L. Treatment of chondromalacia patellae by lateral retinacular release of the patella. Clin Orthop Relat Res 1988;234:145–7.

[17] Lindberg UEP, Lysholm J, Gillquist J. Treatment in patello-femoral arthralgia. Lateral release or conservative treatment? In: Trickey EL, Hertel P, editors. Surgery and arthroscopy of the knee. Berlin; New York: Springer-Verlag; 1986. p. 271.

[18] Van Kampen A, Huiskes R. The three-dimensional tracking pattern of the patella. Thesis, University Nijmegem 1987.

[19] Katchburian MV, Bull AM, Shih YF, et al. Measurement of patellar tracking: assessment and analysis of the literature. Clin Orthop Relat Res 2003;412:241–59.

[20] Maquet P. Biomechanics of the knee. Berlin: Springer-Verlag; 1976.

[21] Brattström H. Shape of the intercondylar groove normally and in recurrent dislocation of the patella. Acta Orthop Scand Suppl 1964;68.

[22] James SL. Chondropalacia of the patella in the adolescent. In: Kennedy JC, editor. The injured adolescent knee. Baltimore (MD): Williams & Wilkens Co; 1979. p. 205–51.

[23] Takai S, Sakakida K, Yamashita F, et al. Rotational alignment of the lower limb in osteoarthritis of the knee. Int Orthop 1985;9:209–16.

[24] Janssen G. Increased medial torsion of the knee joint producing chondromalacia patella. In: Trickey E, Hertel P, editors. Surgery and arthroscopy of the knee, 1984. 2nd edition. Berlin: Springer-Verlag; 1986. p. 263–7.

[25] Laret JL, Moyen B, Galland O, et al. [Morphological types of the lower limbs in femoro-patellar disequilibrium. Analysis in 3 planes]. Acta Orthop Belg 1989;55:347–55 [in French].

[26] Stroud KL, Smith AD, Kruse RW. The relationship between increased femoral anteversion in childhood and patellofemoral pain in adulthood. Orthopaedic Transactions 1989;13:555.

[27] Winson IG, Miranda J, Smith TWD. Anterior knee pain in the post adolescent decade. Acta Orthop Scand 1990;61(Suppl 237):62.

[28] Delgado ED, Schoenecker PL, Rich MM, et al. Treatment of severe torsional malalignment syndrome. J Pediatr Orthop 1996;16:484–8.

[29] Eckhoff DG, Brown AW, Kilcoyne RF, et al. Knee version associated with anterior knee pain. Clin Orthop Relat Res 1997;339:152–5.

[30] Powers CM. The influence of altered lower-extremity kinematics on patellofemoral joint dysfunction: a theoretical perspective. J Orthop Sports Phys Ther 2003;33:639–46.

[31] Lee TQ, Morris G, Csintalan RP. The influence of tibial and femoral rotation on patellofemoral contact area and pressure. J Orthop Sports Phys Ther 2003;33:686–93.

[32] Lang J, Wachsmuth W. Praktische anatomie bein und statik. Berlin: Springer-Verlag; 1972. p. 284.

[33] Yoshioka Y, Siu D, Cooke TDV. The anatomy and functional axes of the femur. J Bone Joint Surg Am 1987;69:873–80.

[34] Yoshioka Y, Cooke TDV. Femoral anteversion: assessment based on functional axes. J Orthop Res 1987;5:86–91.

[35] Murphy SB, Simon SR, Kijewski PK, et al. Femoral anteversion. J Bone Joint Surg Am 1987;69:1169–76.

[36] Yoshioka Y, Siu D, Scudmore RA, et al. Tibial anatomy and functional axes. J Orthop Res 1989;7:132–7.

[37] Conlon T, Garth WF Jr, Lemons JE. Evaluation of the medial soft-tissue restraints of the extensor mechanism of the knee. J Bone Joint Surg Am 1993;75:682–93.

[38] Teitge RA, Faerber W, Des Madryl P, et al. Stress radiographs of the patellofemoral joint. J Bone Joint Surg Am 1996;78:193–203.

[39] Kannus P, Jozsa L. Histopathological changes preceding spontaneous rupture of a tendon. A controlled study of 891 patients. J Bone Joint Surg Am 1991;73:1507–25.

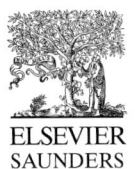

The Management of Recurrent Patellar Dislocation
Jack Andrish, MD

*Department of Orthopaedic Surgery, Cleveland Clinic Foundation, Desk A-41, Cleveland Clinic,
9500 Euclid Avenue, Cleveland, OH 44195, USA*

With the exception of the first paragraph, this chapter was reproduced with permission from Andrish JT. Recurrent patellar dislocation. In: Fulkerson JP, editor. Common patellofemoral problems. Rosemont (IL): American Academy of Orthopedic Surgeons; 2005. p. 43–55.

Acute and chronic trauma, chronic abnormal joint loading conditions, and hemarthroses have been implicated in the development of degenerative joint disease. Patellar instability with acute and recurrent patellar dislocation provides all of these ingredients. It should be no surprise then, that patellofemoral arthritis is ultimately a frequent sequellae to patellar dislocation. Furthermore, although our surgical procedures are most often successful at preventing recurrences of dislocation, they have not been shown to reduce the incidence of patellofemoral arthrosis.

Clark [1] has summarized possible etiologies of patellofemoral arthritis and has presented some evidence to support hypotheses of excessive joint loading and increased duration of joint loading as possible contributors. Patients presenting with recurrent dislocations of the patella typically have variations of anatomy about the knee that predispose to patellar instability. These pathoanatomies may involve variations of lower extremity alignment, patellofemoral alignment, or of trochlear shape. The two most frequent pathoanatomies, trochlear dysplasia and patella alta, have been linked to the development of patellofemoral arthritis, with or without having had a patellar dislocation. Sustaining the additional insult to articular cartilage, which results from the acute trauma of a patellar dislocation, sometimes results in osteochondral fracture, hemarthrosis, and chronic patellar malalignment; patellofemoral arthrosis follows.

This article describes an approach to the treatment of recurrent patellar instability that considers the unique features and expectations of the patient rather than using a generic algorithm. Although an approach that includes an in-depth analysis of the patient's unique pathoanatomy and variations of lower extremity motion is more satisfying than the alternative and would seem to be intellectually defensible [2], its advantages are unsubstantiated. No data exist, however, that suggest that the customized approach described in this article produces results inferior to those achieved by the generic approach, and the intellectual satisfaction is far greater.

To develop a treatment approach that accounts for the unique features of the patient who has recurrent patellar dislocations, an understanding of how neuromuscular, ligamentous, and morphologic variations of the lower extremity contribute to patellar stability or instability is required. Treatment can then be designed to address the pathologies of form and function rather than to compensate for those abnormalities by creating secondary pathoanatomies.

Epidemiology and natural history

In a prospective study of a Kaiser Health Plan population, individuals in their second decade of life had the highest incidence of acute patellar dislocation, with 69% of all dislocations that occurred in a year affecting these individuals. The overall risk for members of this health plan for all ages was 7 per 100,000 per year, but the risk for those between the ages of 10 to 19 years was 31 per 100,000 per year, with a nearly equal distribution among girls and American Academy

E-mail address: andrisj@ccf.org

of Orthopaedic Surgeons boys (33 per 100,000 per years versus 30 per 100,000 per year, respectively) [3].

Female sex, a family history of patellar instability, and a history of patellar subluxation or dislocation have been associated with higher risk of subsequent dislocation [3,4]. Furthermore, the degree of trauma associated with the first dislocation is an important indicator of subsequent dislocation [3]. Fithian and associates [3] note that in patients who have MRI-documented disruption of the medial retinaculum and the medial patellofemoral ligament (MPFL), the incidence of subsequent patellar dislocation was lower than in patients without retinacular injury. This finding is understandable if one considers that patellar dislocation in the absence of MPFL trauma may be indicative of coexisting patellofemoral dysplasia. Crosby and Insall [5] reported that episodes of patellar subluxation/dislocation decreased with time, and the incidence of patellofemoral osteoarthritis was low and not related to the frequency of dislocations.

Biomechanics of patellar instability

Patellar motion is affected by the complex interaction of muscles, ligaments, bone morphology, and lower extremity alignment [6,7]. The retinacular patellofemoral ligaments are important stabilizers of the patella, and, in particular, the MPFL is the primary soft-tissue restraint to lateral translation of the patella during the initial 20° to 30° of knee flexion [8–12]. This ligament is most taut in full extension, with the quadriceps contracted, and assists in guiding the patella into the trochlea during the early stages of flexion [13]. Amis and associates [13] and Senavongse and associates [14] demonstrated that the least resistance to lateral translation of the patella occurs at 20° of flexion, with increasing resistance occurring with further extension and flexion. Once engaged in the trochlea, the patellofemoral joint compression provided by the increasing force vectors of the quadriceps and patellar tendons, combined with patellofemoral joint geometry, provides the major effect on stability as knee flexion progresses [15–17]. While the patella is tracking within the trochlea, the slope of the lateral facet of the trochlea provides the main resistance to lateral patellar translation [18,19]. Studies have been conducted on the influence of the musculature and the vastus medialis obliquus (VMO) in particular on knee stability [20–22]. The evidence supporting the VMO as a major determinant in patellofemoral stability is controversial, but as with the retinacular patellofemoral ligaments, the VMO exerts its greatest influence on patellar alignment during the initial stages of knee flexion [22,23].

Several studies have examined the influence of lower extremity alignment on patellar instability [17,24–27]. Fithian and associates [12] demonstrated, however, that lower extremity and patellofemoral alignment cannot by themselves produce an episode of patellar dislocation without the coexistence of an insufficiency of the soft-tissue restraints by hyperelasticity or injury.

Patient history

Chronic recurrent dislocations and subluxations of the patella are often more disabling to the patient than isolated ligamentous instability of the knee, and they are more disabling than instability associated with injury to the anterior cruciate ligament (ACL). The difference is that instability that is the result of a torn ACL is typically symptomatic during sport activity. Although this is a significant concern for the active individual, only 15% to 30% of patients who have torn ACLs experience instability symptoms with activities of daily living [28–31]. Conversely, patellar instability is typically associated with the knee giving way unexpectedly with minimal trauma during activities of daily living. This sometimes results in significant secondary injuries from falls, and these patients are frequently extremely apprehensive.

Another important distinction to be made from the history is the patient's perception of the relative importance of the pain. Patellar dislocations are painful, but the pain is secondary to the event. The patient who reports knee pain as the primary problem, with patellar instability events as secondary ("My knee hurts all of the time, and sometimes it gives out on me") is viewed differently from the patient whose instability is the primary reason for the consultation ("My knee hurts, but the main reason I am here is that when my patella slips out, the pain is severe"). Good orthopedic tools exist to manage instability and the pain that is secondary to the events resulting from instability, but treatment of chronic knee pain or chronic pain associated with patellar instability becomes more difficult. There are multiple causes of chronic knee pain, and not all are structural in nature [32].

Age at onset and the magnitude of trauma eliciting the patellar dislocation are important. If a significant trauma such as a contact injury in sport (valgus, external rotation of the tibia versus a direct lateralizing blow to the patella) is the first event that produced a patellar dislocation. If the soft-tissue and joint reaction to this trauma is severe, it is likely that the inherent stability of the patella was normal at the time of injury and that closed or open management will be successful unless a significant osteochondral fracture complicates the outcome. On the other hand, if the event was trivial, such as a minor twist or pivot, then it is likely that the patient has one or a combination of pathoanatomies (dynamic or static) that predisposed the knee to the first episode and will contribute to recurrent episodes. In these patients, closed management is frequently insufficient, and even surgical management may result in failure unless the unique features that allowed for the dislocation are adequately addressed [33].

Physical examination

Physical examination of the patient who has chronic recurrent dislocations of the patella involves an awareness of the whole individual. The patient may be apprehensive. The gait may be somewhat unusual because these patients often use innovative adaptive mechanisms to avoid further episodes. Typically, the patient shows significant apprehension with attempted palpation of the patella, especially with assessment of medial and lateral patellar translation. The examination may be divided into assessments made with the patient standing, walking, sitting, lying supine, lying prone, and lying on the side.

Standing

James and associates [34] coined the term "miserable malalignment" syndrome. This finding consists of a kneeing-in posture, or "squinting" patellae, coexisting with proximal tibia vara, medial femoral torsion, an increased Q angle, and either hyperpronation of the foot, external tibial torsion, or both [34]. Although this lower extremity posture is often found in patients who have anterior knee pain, it may be part of a series of anatomic variances associated with but not necessarily causative of patellar instability.

Walking

Not all abnormalities that contribute to patellar instability are static deformities. The dynamics of the patient's gait may demonstrate pathomechanics unique to the individual that predispose to patellar malalignment and instability. The gait most often associated with patellofemoral dysfunction is the kneeing-in gait. This is frequently described as being secondary to medial femoral torsion (femoral anteversion), but it can just as easily be secondary to external tibial torsion, hyperpronation of the foot, or some combination of the three [35]. Kneeing-in is significant because the internal rotation and valgus thrust generates an external rotation moment about the knee with a resultant lateral force on the patella [17]. Although this gait is most frequently associated with the static deformities described previously, it may be dynamically induced by altered neuromotor coordination, as in spasticity, or it may be a result of instability of the core musculature of the back, abdomen, and hip [36,37].

Sitting

With the patient in the seated position with the knees at the edge of the examining table, assessment of the relative height of the patellae may reveal patella alta or patella baja [38]. The Q angle obtained while the patient is sitting may be more meaningful than when the patient is lying supine because most often the patella is centered in the trochlea at 30° to 90° of flexion [39–41]. With the knee in full extension, however, the patella may be laterally positioned, thus giving the illusion of a normal Q angle. To measure the Q angle in the sitting position, drop a plumb line from the center of the patella. The line should bisect the tibial tuberosity. If the tuberosity is lateral to this line, an abnormally increased Q angle exists [40,41].

Active knee extension may elicit patellofemoral crepitus, which is suggestive of articular surface injury or degeneration. An extensor lag may signify significant weakness of the quadriceps mechanism, or it may be the result of severe patellar instability with obligatory subluxation or even dislocation with active extension. The J sign or J-tracking is frequently associated with patella alta or trochlear dysplasia.

Medial subluxations or even dislocations of the patella may be difficult to detect without stress radiography, although using the Fulkerson [42] relocation test can be helpful. In this test, the knee is passively supported in extension, and the patella is gently subluxated medially. Then the knee is gently flexed while allowing the patella to relocate. If this maneuver results in sudden pain or apprehension and especially if the patient relates the sensation to his or her presenting symptoms, the diagnosis of medial patellar subluxation should be considered. Finally, with the patient in the sitting position, the upper extremities can be examined for signs of generalized laxity [43,44].

Lying supine

With the patient in the supine position, the examiner can observe, palpate, and test for knee stability and for joint motion and irritability (in the hip and in the knee). The relative girth and development of the quadriceps and asymmetric or significant atrophy of the VMO may be observed. Effusion may be detected from observation alone, but palpation further quantifies the extent. Palpation also detects areas of retinacular tenderness, and patellofemoral compression may provoke crepitus or pain. Patellar mobility is assessed with the knee fully extended and then with the knee flexed 30° [45–48]. Significant apprehension with passive subluxation is indicative of clinical subluxations. Hypermobility of the patella may confirm the clinical suspicion of patellar subluxations and dislocations, whereas the absence of hypermobility may be even more meaningful because it suggests other possibilities for symptoms of giving way. The presence of a firm end point when lateral stress is applied to the patella, combined with limited translation (two quadrants or less), mitigates against the diagnosis of patellar instability [33]. The supine examination should include general assessment and documentation of collateral, capsular, and cruciate stability.

Lying prone

The prone position is best used for detection of femoral and tibial torsion and quadriceps contracture. This position allows maintenance of hip extension while flexing the knee to observe the heel-to-buttock distance. Involuntary pelvic tilt and hip flexion during this maneuver indicates tightness of the rectus femoris (Ely test) [37]. Inability to fully flex the knee may indicate quadriceps contracture or (painful) internal derangement of the knee.

The transmalleolar axis of the ankle is most relevant to tibial torsion (normally externally rotated 15°), whereas measurement of the amount of internal and external rotation of the hip reveals abnormalities of femoral torsion. The foot position also suggests variations in tibial torsion, but it is important to account for pes planus because the abducted foot position may be confused with external tibial torsion.

Side lying

This final position is best used to detect contracture of the iliotibial tract (Ober's test). In the Ober test, the knee and hip are flexed. Holding the knee in flexion, the hip is abducted and then extended (holding the knee flexed). The hip is then allowed to adduct. A tight iliotibial band prevents adduction of the hip in this position. The side lying position also can be used to detect (iatrogenic) medial patellar subluxation as described by Nonweiler and DeLee [49].

Radiographic findings

Many authors have described variations in patellar alignment and patellofemoral morphology that may relate to patellar instability [39,50–52], specifically, those that could be implicated as risk factors for dislocation. Although the order of importance varies among the studies, patella alta and trochlear dysplasia have been identified consistently as important factors associated with recurrent patellar dislocations [39,50,53–55]. Other factors are patellar tilt and increased lateralization of the tibial tuberosity in relation to the trochlear groove [56,57]. Although Dejour and associates [50] believed that patellar tilt was indicative of quadriceps dysplasia, Arendt and associates [33] and Beasley and Vidal [58] related this to insufficiency of the MPFL, which some have implicated as the essential lesion involved in recurrent patellar instability.

Radiographs remain important in the evaluation of patients who have patellar instability. Although CT has been viewed as a more sensitive indicator of patellar malalignment because of the ability to obtain axial images in the more provocative degrees of knee flexion (at and near full extension), Murray and associates [59] demonstrated that true lateral radiographs provide similar information. Specifically, the anterior posterior (AP) view provides an assessment of femoral-tibial alignment and arthrosis, and the lateral view provides an assessment of patellar height, tilt, subluxation, and arthrosis [60]. The depth of the trochlear sulcus and variations of dysplasia of the distal femur are readily identified. The axial view, as described by Laurin and associates [61] and by Merchant and associates [62], adds to our understanding of trochlear shape and patellar position. Patella alta is frequently associated with patellar instability; therefore, assessment by radiography is important. Although the Insall-Salvati index and the measurement described by Caton and associates are popular measurements of the patellar height, the index described by Blackburne and Peel is more reproducible [60].

CT provides important views of patellofemoral alignment and congruence in the early stages of knee flexion, but MRI can provide the same information and has the added advantage of demonstrating the articular cartilage [19,52,57,63,64]. Staubli and associates [64] demonstrated that the contour of the articular cartilage of the patellofemoral joint does not always follow the contour of the subchondral bone. Therefore, it is possible for CT images to seem to show patellofemoral incongruence when the MRI scan reveals true articular congruence. Furthermore, recent demonstrations of dynamic MRI suggest additional advantages in the evaluation of patellofemoral dysfunction [65]. Nevertheless, the extensive database of CT measurements and the efficiency of time and expense for CT versus MRI justify its continued use in the evaluation of patellofemoral alignment.

Historic treatment options and outcomes

Nonsurgical

Nonsurgical management of patellar dislocations has resulted in redislocation rates of 15% to 44% with persistent symptoms of anterior knee pain, instability, and limitations of activity affecting more than 50% of patients [66–68]. Although nonsurgical management protocols vary widely, those including early mobilization have resulted in poorer outcomes [68,69].

Surgical

The literature describes more than 100 different surgical approaches for recurrent patellar dislocation; [70–75] however, variations in reporting and study design make comparisons among these studies almost impossible. Traditionally, surgical regimens have been one of three types: proximal realignment, distal realignment, or combined combination of the two. In studies comparing efficacy of proximal versus distal alignment, distal shows no benefit over proximal [76]. Lateral retinacular release as an isolated procedure for patellar instability has been shown to have inferior outcomes [76,77].

Finally, studies comparing surgical and nonsurgical treatment of patellar instability have failed to show superior long-term clinical results with surgical treatment [78,79]. Some studies of surgical treatment have shown an increased risk of developing patellofemoral arthrosis despite the reduction in dislocations after surgery [80–85].

My preferred management

The knee is a coupled mechanical system in which a change to any one part of the system affects the other parts of the system [86]. For example, a tibial tuberosity transfer may affect joint loading within the patellofemoral and tibiofemoral joints. Medial transfer of the tibial tuberosity increases joint loading within the medial tibio-femoral compartment and the medial facet of the patellofemoral joint and inducing variable changes within the lateral tibiofemoral compartment [87]. Therefore, medialization of the tibial tuberosity should be used cautiously in the varus knee and, if possible, avoided in the medial menisectomized knee. Anteriorization of the tibial tuberosity decreases patellofemoral contact pressures in general; however, the transfer of those forces to a more proximal location on the patella may result in increased loading in those areas [88]. Therefore, anteriorization and anteromedialization of the tibial tuberosity should be used only after recognizing the patellar wear patterns, and they should be avoided when the resultant loads are increased over areas of severe articular cartilage degeneration [89].

Nonsurgical

Despite the disability that results from recurrent patellar dislocations, persistence with nonsurgical treatment is warranted when the dislocations are isolated or infrequent, not habitual or obligatory, and, most importantly, when the existing patellar mechanics are able to accommodate the rehabilitation process. When the patella dislocates painfully with each attempt at active knee extension, it is often better to perform the realignment first and then begin pelvi-femoral rehabilitation once the patella is well aligned and stable.

A rehabilitation program may be successful in the patient who has a history of a series of isolated patellar dislocations that occasionally affect work or play but in whom there are no overriding mechanical or intra-articular reasons to proceed immediately with a surgical procedure [90]. Pelvifemoral rehabilitation is based on a philosophy of providing core stability through strengthening of the anatomic core musculature (hip, abdomen, back) in addition to the traditional quadriceps progressive resistance exercises [91]. Although the VMO is an important component of patellar stability, its role as the main dynamic stabilizer has been overstated [22,23,92–94]. Weakness of the anatomic core musculature may allow for excessive medial femoral rotation and knee valgus, which may contribute or predispose to patellar dislocation or subluxation [17]. Therefore, we initiate and monitor the rehabilitation process for compliance and outcome, and, most importantly, we emphasize to the patient and his or her family that the exercise program is to be continued over the long term to ensure continuing optimal function.

For patients who desire an orthosis, there are several good choices, although the literature lacks evidence-based support [95–97]. For uncomplicated patellar subluxation, I prefer the simple Neoprene J brace. For the patient who has significant instability symptoms and who wishes to remain active in sports, and especially if there is a component of hypermobility, the TruePull brace (Donjoy Ortho, Vista, CA) designed by Fulkerson has been well tolerated. For the patient who has a significant J sign, the Breg patellar tendon orthosis (PTO Neoprene) (Breg Inc., Vista, CA) offers at least a theoretic advantage by exerting a restraining force against lateral displacement, which is greater in extension than in flexion. If a brace is used in the nonsurgical treatment of patellar instability, the brace should be considered an adjunct to, not a substitute for, the rehabilitation process.

Surgical

Rather than describing common surgical procedures used for the treatment of patellar instability, I prefer to abandon the "procedure" mentality in favor of an "identify and address the pathoanatomy" approach. I consider a surgical procedure based on whether it addresses an existing pathoanatomy that allows or provokes episodes of patellar subluxation or dislocation. It is possible to identify the anatomic variances unique to the individual (Box 1) [63,98]. My first principle in designing a treatment for patellar instability is to individualize, customize, and normalize. My preference is to correct the offending pathoanatomy, not to create a secondary pathoanatomy to compensate for the primary pathoanatomy. In choosing a procedure, I consider the risk versus the benefit of the individual procedures. Soft-tissue proximal realignment has been shown to be as effective as distal realignment in the treatment of patellar instability [76].

Box 1. Pathoanatomies of patellar instability

Trochlear dysplasia
Patella alta
Increased "Q" angle
Increased TT:TG distance
Tibial tuberosity:trochlear groove
Medial patellofemoral ligament
  insufficiency
VMO hypoplasia/dysplasia
Vastus lateralis dominance
Contracture
Lateral retinaculum
I-T band
Rectus femoris or Vastus lateralis
  Congenital patellar dislocations
  Obligatory patellar dislocations
Lower extremity malalignment
Torsion
  Femur, medial
  Tibia, lateral
Genu valgum
Gait
Valgus thrust
Valgus/internal rotation thrust
Excessive medial rotation of femur with
  increased external rotation torque of
  knee
  Medial femoral torsion
  External tibial torsion
  Excessive foot pronation
  "Core" instability

Data from Andrish JT. Recurrent patellar dislocation. In: Fulkerson JP, editor. Common patellofemoral problems. Monograph series #29. Rosemont (IL): American Academy of Orthopaedic Surgeons; 2005. p. 43–55.

This approach requires careful and thorough patient evaluation before surgery, including assessment of lower extremity alignment, patellar position and mobility, quadriceps balance, and gait. It also requires a careful radiographic assessment of patellofemoral joint morphology and alignment. I then plan for the method of anesthesia to be used. I prefer to use selective epidural anesthesia or local anesthesia and monitored anesthesia control because it allows the patient to actively extend the knee on command during the surgery. This method is useful when rebalancing the extensor mechanism and is invaluable in patients who have obligatory patellar dislocations that occur with active knee extension or with knee flexion. It is desirable and helpful for patients with a prominent J sign and lateral pull.

After identification of the pathoanatomies, I consider the risk versus the benefit of the surgical correction of these components. The correction of bone shape or alignment by osteotomy can be compelling, but the use of this procedure should be weighed against potential risks of overcorrection, undercorrection, delayed union or nonunion, late fracture, and pathologic changes in joint loading [25,86,87,99,100]. Nevertheless, for some patients the most appropriate surgical tool is an osteotomy.

Soft-tissue realignment or reconstruction may be perceived by some as safer, but it requires a high level of surgical expertise and experience [3], and the potential exists to make the repair/ reconstruction too tight. The goal of realignment of the extensor mechanism is to reestablish the balance of forces that results in patellar stability while maintaining physiologic motion. Stability should not be achieved through overconstraint. Although I recognize the importance of the medial retinacular ligaments and the MPFL in particular in enabling the consistent and safe engagement of the patella into the femoral trochlea during the initial 10° to 30° of knee flexion, I do not depend on the MPFL to hold the patella in place. If I use that philosophy (and I have in the past), the potential exists to make the repair/ reconstruction too tight. This may result in pain, stiffness, and potential patellofemoral joint overload. The other risk with patellar realignments that rely too heavily on MPFL repair or reconstruction to hold the patella in place while other pathoanatomies affecting alignment are not corrected is the eventual stretching and subsequent incompetence of the procedure. Based on these factors, I prefer to make the medial repair/ reconstruction one of the last components of the procedure. After realigning the patella through some combination of osteotomy of the tibial tuberosity, distal femur, or lengthening of the lateral retinaculum or quadriceps components (vastus lateralis, rectus femoris), the MPFL is identified and retensioned or reconstructed as needed.

Although proximal patellar realignment has been described, I will elaborate on a few details. The lateral retinaculum contributes to lateral and medial patellar stability [9,101]. The creation of iatrogenic medial instability of the patella is uncommon but not rare [38,100,102]. To release the lateral retinaculum in the presence of patellar instability risks further destabilization of an unstable joint [3,14]. If the lateral retinaculum is a pathoanatomy by virtue of contracture, then lengthening is preferred over release. Larson and associates [103] described a method of lateral retinacular lengthening that helps avoid the potential complication of medial patellar subluxation. In some patients, symptomatic patellar hypermobility has responded to reconstruction of a previously released lateral retinaculum [104].

Surgically balancing the actions of the vastus lateralis and the VMO can be a challenge because the VMO commonly is dysplastic. It can be severely atrophic or more vertically oriented rather than oblique. VMO advancement traditionally has been included in proximal realignment, but advancement over the patella does little to increase its mechanical effectiveness. Detachment of the VMO to advance it distally over the patella can impair its effectiveness by reducing the obliquity of its fibers. It is more advisable to advance the posteromedial corner of the VMO tendon as described by Ahmad and associates [105] to increase its obliquity and mechanical advantage. That said, the vastus lateralis is generally a larger muscle than the VMO with a total cross-sectional area of the quadriceps of 40% compared with 25% for the VMO [92]. Also, a less often described portion of the vastus lateralis is comparable to a vastus lateralis obliquus. When the lateral retinaculum is lengthened rather than released, this oblique portion of the lateralis may be released, and, if necessary, a portion of the lateralis tendon can be lengthened (with suture repair after a 1- to 3-cm lengthening) to effect quadriceps balance [106]. This may be necessary in some cases of severe lateral pull with subluxation/ dislocation in active extension and especially in congenital and obligatory dislocations associated with contracture of the vastus lateralis [107,108].

[19] the lateral trochlear inclination. Initial experience. Radiology 2000;216:582–5.
[20] Neptune RR, Wright IC, van den Bogert AJ. The influence of orthotic devices and vastus medialis strength and timing on patellofemoral loads during running. Clin Biomech 2000;15:611–8.
[21] Raimondo RA, Ahmad CS, Blankevoort L, et al. Patellar stabilization: a quantitative evaluation of the vastus medialis obliquus muscle. Orthopedics 1998;21:791–5.
[22] Sakai N, Luo ZP, Rand JA, et al. The influence of weakness in the vastus medialis oblique muscle on the patellofemoral joint: an in vitro biomechanical study. Clin Biomech 2000;15:335–9.
[23] Goh JCH, Lee PYC, Bose K. A cadaver study of the function of the oblique part of vastus medialis. J Bone Joint Surg Br 1995;77:225–31.
[24] Livingston LA. The quadriceps angle: a review of the literature. J Orthop Sports Phys Ther 1998;28:105–9.
[25] Mizuno Y, Kumagai M, Mattessich SM, et al. Q-angle influences tibiofemoral and patellofemoral kinematics. J Orthop Res 2001;19:834–40.
[26] Post WR, Teitge R, Amis A. Patellofemoral malalignment: looking beyond the viewbox. Clin Sports Med 2002;21:521–46.
[27] Sanfridsson J, Arnbjornsson A, Friden T, et al. Femorotibial rotation and the Q-angle related to the dislocating patella. Acta Radiol 2001;42:218–24.
[28] Buckley SL, Barrack RL, Alexander AH. The natural history of conservatively treated partial anterior cruciate ligament tears. Am J Sports Med 1989;17:221–5.
[29] Daniel DM, Stone ML, Dobson BE, et al. Fate of the ACL-injured patient: a prospective outcome study. Am J Sports Med 1994;22:632–44.
[30] McDaniel WJ, Dameron TB. Untreated ruptures of the anterior cruciate ligament. J Bone Joint Surg Am 1980;62:696–704.
[31] Noyes FR, Mooar PA, Matthews DS, et al. The symptomatic anterior cruciate-deficient knee: part I. The long-term functional disability in athletically active individuals. J Bone Joint Surg Am 1983;65:154–62.
[32] Dye SF. Patellofemoral pain current concepts: an overview. Sports Medicine and Arthroscopy Review 2001;9:264–72.
[33] Arendt EA, Fithian DC, Cohen E. Current concepts of lateral patella dislocation. Clin Sports Med 2002;21:499–519.
[34] James SL, Bates BT, Osternig LR. Injuries to runners. Am J Sports Med 1978;6:40–50.
[35] James SL. Running injuries to the knee. J Am Acad Orthop Surg 1995;3:309–18.
[36] Hutchinson MR, Ireland ML. Knee injuries in female athletes. Sports Med 1995;19:288–302.
[37] Zeller BL, McCrory JL, Kibler B, et al. Differences in kinematics and electromyographic activity between men and women during the single-legged squat. Am J Sports Med 2003;31:449–56.
[38] Hughston JC, Deese M. Medial subluxation of the patella as a complication of lateral retinacular release. Am J Sports Med 1988;16:383–8.
[39] Atkin DM, Fithian DC, Marangi KS, et al. Characteristics of patients with primary acute lateral patellar dislocation and their recovery within the first 6 months of injury. Am J Sports Med 2000;28:472–9.
[40] Kolowich PA, Paulos LE, Rosenberg TD, et al. Lateral release of the patella: indications and contraindications. Am J Sports Med 1990;18:359–65.
[41] Post WR, Fulkerson JP. Distal realignment of the patellofemoral joint: indications, effects, results and recommendations. Orthop Clin North Am 1992;23:631–43.
[42] Fulkerson JP. Anterolateralization of the tibial tubercle. Tech Orthop 1997;12:165–9.
[43] DeLee JC, Drez D. Etiology of injury to the foot and ankle. In: Stevenson A, editor. 2nd edition. Orthopaedic sports medicine: principles and practice, vol. 2. Philadelphia: Saunders; 2003. p. 2224–74.
[44] Steiner ME. Hypermobility and knee injuries. The Physician and Sports Medicine 1987;15:159–65.
[45] Fithian DC, Mishra DK, Balen PF, et al. Instrumented measurement of patellar mobility. Am J Sports Med 1995;23:607–15.
[46] Skalley TC, Terry GC, Teitge RA. The quantitative measurement of normal passive medial and lateral patellar motion limits. Am J Sports Med 1993;21:728–32.
[47] Tanner SM, Garth WP, Soileau R, et al. A modified test for patellar instability: the biomechanical basis. Clin J Sport Med 2003;13:327–38.
[48] Teitge RA, Faerber W, Des Madryl P, et al. Stress radiographs of the patellofemoral joint. J Bone Joint Surg Am 1996;78:193–203.
[49] Nonweiler DE, DeLee JC. The diagnosis and treatment of medial subluxation of the patella after lateral retinacular release. Am J Sports Med 1994;22:680–6.
[50] Dejour H, Walch G, Nove-Josserand L, et al. Factors of patellar instability: an anatomic radiographic study. Knee Surg Sports Traumatol Arthrosc 1994;2:19–26.
[51] Dupont JY, Guier CA. Comparison of three standard radiologic techniques for screening of patellar subluxations. Clin Sports Med 2002;21:389–401.
[52] Kujala UM, Osterman K, Kormano M, et al. Patellofemoral relationships in recurrent patellar dislocation. J Bone Joint Surg Br 1989;71:788–92.
[53] Dejour H, Walch G, Neyret PH, et al. Dysplasia of the femoral trochlea. Rev Chir Orthop Reparatrice Appar Mot 1990;76:45–54.
[54] Galland O, Walch G, Dejour H, et al. An anatomical and radiological study of the femoropatellar articulation. Surg Radiol Anat 1990;12:119–25.

[55] Lancourt JE, Cristini JA. Patella alta and patella infera: their etiological role in patellar dislocation, chondromalacia, and apophysitis of the tibial tubercle. J Bone Joint Surg Am 1975;57:1112–5.

[56] Nove-Josserand L, Dejour D. Quadriceps dysplasia and patellar tilt in objective patellar instability. Rev Chir Orthop Reparatrice Appar Mot 1995;81: 497–504.

[57] Tsujimoto K, Kurosaka M, Yoshiya S, et al. Radiographic and computed tomographic analysis of the position of the tibial tubercle in recurrent dislocation and subluxation of the patella. Am J Knee Surg 2000;13:83–8.

[58] Beasley LS, Vidal AF. Traumatic patellar dislocation in children and adolescents: treatment update and literature review. Curr Opin Pediatr 2004;16: 29–36.

[59] Murray TF, Dupont JY, Fulkerson JP. Axial and lateral radiographs in evaluating patellofemoral malalignment. Am J Sports Med 1999;27: 580–4.

[60] Berg EE, Mason SL, Lucas MJ. Patellar height ratios: a comparison of four measurement methods. Am J Sports Med 1996;24:218–21.

[61] Laurin CA, Dussault R, Levesque HP. The tangential x-ray investigation of the patellofemoral joint: X-ray technique, American academy of orthopaedic surgeons diagnostic criteria and their interpretation. Clin Orthop 1979;144:16–26.

[62] Merchant AC, Mercer RL, Jacobsen RH, et al. Roentgenographic analysis of patellofemoral congruence. J Bone Joint Surg Am 1974;56:1391–6.

[63] Kobayashi T, Fujikawa K. Theoretical use of 3D CT to predict method of patella realignment. Knee 2003;10:135–8.

[64] Staubli HU, Durrenmatt U, Porcellini B, et al. Anatomy and surface geometry of the patellofemoral joint in the axial plane. J Bone Joint Surg Br 1999;81:452–8.

[65] von Eisenhart-Rothe R, Siebert M, Bringmann C, et al. A new in vivo technique for determination of 3D kinematics and contact areas of the patellofemoral and tibio-femoral joint. J Biomech 2004;27: 927–34.

[66] Hawkins RJ, Bell RH, Anisette G. Acute patellar dislocations: the natural history. Am J Sports Med 1986;14:117–20.

[67] Tuxoe JI, Teir M, Winge S, et al. A medial patellofemoral ligament: a dissection study. Knee Surg Sports Traumatol Arthrosc 2002;10:138–40.

[68] Harilainen A, Myllynen P. Operative treatment in acute patellar dislocation: radiological predisposing factors, diagnosis and results. Am J Knee Surg 1988;1:178–85.

[69] Maenpaa H, Lehto MU. Patellar dislocation: the long-term results of nonoperative management in 100 patients. Am J Sports Med 1997;25:213–7.

[70] Brown DE, Alexander AH, Lightman DM. The elmslie-trillat procedure: evaluation in patellar dislocation and subluxation. Am J Sports Med 1984;12:104–9.

[71] Fondren FB, Goldner JL, Bassett FH. Recurrent dislocation of the patella treated by the modified roux-goldthwait procedure. J Bone Joint Surg Am 1985;67:993–1005.

[72] Letts RM, Davidson D, Beaule P. Semitendinosus tenodesis for repair of recurrent dislocation of the patella in children. J Pediatr Orthop 1999;19:742–7.

[73] Madigan R, Wissinger HA, Donaldson WF. Preliminary experience with a method of quadricepsplasty in recurrent subluxation of the patella. J Bone Joint Surg Am 1975;57:600–7.

[74] Myers P, Williams A, Dodds R, et al. The three-in-one proximal and distal soft tissue patellar realignment procedure: results and its place in the management of patellofemoral instability. Am J Sports Med 1999;27:575–9.

[75] Wootton JR, Cross MR, Wood DG. Patellofemoral malalignment: a report of 68 cases treated by proximal and distal patellofemoral reconstruction. Injury 1990;21:169–73.

[76] Aglietti P, Buzzi R, De Biase P, et al. Surgical treatment of recurrent dislocation of the patella. Clin Orthop 1994;308:8–17.

[77] Fulkerson JP, Schutzer SF, Ramsby GR, et al. Computerized tomography of the patellofemoral joint before and after lateral release or realignment. Arthroscopy 1987;3:19–24.

[78] Nikku R, Nietosvaara Y, Kallio PE, et al. Operative versus closed treatment of primary dislocation of the patella. Acta Orthop Scand 1997;68: 419–23.

[79] Powers JA. Natural history of recurrent dislocation of the patella. Clin Orthop 1976;119:281.

[80] Arnbjornsson A, Eglund N, Rydling O, et al. The natural history of recurrent dislocation of the patella: long-term results of conservative and operative treatment. J Bone Joint Surg Br 1992;74: 140–2.

[81] Hampson WGJ, Hill P. Late results of transfer of the tibial tubercle for recurrent dislocation of the patella. J Bone Joint Surg Br 1975;57:209–13.

[82] Juliusson R, Markhede G. A modified hauser procedure for recurrent dislocation of the patella: a long-term follow-up study with special reference to osteoarthritis. Arch Orthop Trauma Surg 1984; 103:42–6.

[83] Maenpaa H, Lehto MU. Patellofemoral osteoarthritis after patellar dislocation. Clin Orthop 1997;339:156–62.

[84] Nakagawa K, Wada Y, Minamide M, et al. Deterioration of long-term clinical results after the elmslie-trillat procedure for dislocation of the patella. J Bone Joint Surg Br 2002;84:861–4.

[85] Shellock FG. Effect of a patellar realignment brace on patients with patellar subluxation and dislocation: evaluation with kinematic magnetic resonance imaging. Am J Sports Med 2000;28:131–3.

[86] Kuroda R, Kambic H, Valdevit A, et al. Articular cartilage contact pressure after tibial tuberosity transfer. Am J Sports Med 2001;29:403–9.

[87] Huberti HH, Hayes WC. Patellofemoral contact pressures: the influence of Q-angle and tendofemoral contact. J Bone Joint Surg Am 1984;66:715–24.

[88] Ahmed AM, Burke DL, Hyder A. Force analysis of the patellar mechanism. J Orthop Res 1987;5:69–85.

[89] Pidoriano AJ, Weinstein RN, Buuck DA, et al. Correlation of patellar articular lesions with results from anteromedial tibial tubercle transfer. Am J Sports Med 1997;25:533–7.

[90] Wilk KE, Davies GJ, Mangine RE, et al. Patellofemoral disorders: a classification system and clinical guidelines for nonoperative rehabilitation. J Orthop Sports Phys Ther 1998;28:307–22.

[91] Steinkamp LA, Dillingham MF, Markel MD, et al. Biomechanical considerations in patellofemoral joint rehabilitation. Am J Sports Med 1993;21:438–44.

[92] Farahmand F, Senavongse W, Amis A. Quantitative study of the quadriceps muscles and trochlear groove geometry related to instability of the patellofemoral joint. J Orthop Res 1998;16:136–43.

[93] Grabiner MD, Koh TJ, Miller GF. Fatigue rates of vastus medialis oblique and vastus lateralis during static and dynamic knee extension. J Orthop Res 1991;9:391–7.

[94] Lieb FJ, Perry J. Quadriceps function: an anatomical and mechanical study using amputated limbs. J Bone Joint Surg Am 1968;50:1535–48.

[95] Muhle C, Brinkmann G, Skaf A, et al. Effect of a patellar realignment brace on patients with patellar subluxation and dislocation. Am J Sports Med 1999;27:350–3.

[96] Palumbo PM. Dynamic patellar brace: a new orthosis in the management of patellofemoral disorders. Am J Sports Med 1981;9:45–9.

[97] Shellock FG. Effect of a patella-stabilizing brace on lateral subluxation of the patella. Am J Knee Surg 2000;13:137–42.

[98] Harilainen A, Sandelin J. Prospective long-term results of operative treatment in primary dislocation of the patella. Knee Surg Sports Traumatol Arthrosc 1993;1:100–3.

[99] Godde S, Rupp S, Dienst M, et al. Fracture of the proximal tibia six months after Fulkerson osteotomy. J Bone Joint Surg Br 2001;83:832–3.

[100] Teitge RA. Treatment of complications of patellofemoral joint surgery. Oper Tech Sports Med 1994;2:317–34.

[101] Luo ZP, Sakai N, Rand JA, et al. Tensile stress of the lateral patellofemoral ligament during knee motion. Am J Knee Surg 1997;10:139–44.

[102] Ahmad CS, Sinicropi SM, Su B, et al. Congenital medial dislocation of the patella. Orthopedics 2003;26:189–90.

[103] Larson RL, Cabaud HE, Slocum DB, et al. The patellar compression syndrome: surgical treatment by lateral retinacular release. Clin Orthop 1978;134:158–67.

[104] Johnson DP, Wakeley C. Reconstruction of the lateral patellar retinaculum following lateral release: a case report. Knee Surg Sports Traumatol Arthrosc 2002;10:361–3.

[105] Ahmad CS, Stein BES, Matuz D, et al. Immediate surgical repair of the medial patellar stabilizers for acute patellar dislocation: a review of eight cases. Am J Sports Med 2000;22:804–10.

[106] Hughston JC. Reconstruction of the extensor mechanism for subluxating patella. J Sports Med 1972;1:6–13.

[107] Eilert RE. Dysplasia of the patellofemoral joint in children. Am J Knee Surg 1999;12:114–9.

[108] Lai KA, Shen WJ, Lin CJ, et al. Vastus lateralis fibrosis in habitual patella dislocation. Acta Orthop Scand 2000;71:394–8.

[109] Avikainen VJ, Nikku RK, Seppanen-Lehmonen TK. Adductor magnus tenodesis for patellar dislocation. Clin Orthop 1993;297:12–6.

[110] Deie M, Ochi M, Sumen Y, et al. Reconstruction of the medial patellofemoral ligament for the treatment of habitual or recurrent dislocation of the patella in children. J Bone Joint Surg Br 2003;85:887–90.

[111] Gomes JLE. Medial patellofemoral ligament reconstruction for recurrent dislocation of the patella: a preliminary report. Arthroscopy 1992;8:335–40.

[112] Muneta T, Sekiya I, Tsuchiya M, et al. A technique for reconstruction of the medial patellofemoral ligament. Clin Orthop 1999;359:151–5.

[113] Nomura E, Inoue M. Surgical technique and rationale for medial patellofemoral ligament reconstruction for recurrent patellar dislocation. Arthroscopy 2003;19:1–9.

[114] Hughston JC, Flandry F, Brinker MR, et al. Surgical correction of medial subluxation of the patella. Am J Sports Med 1996;24:486–91.

[115] Neyret Ph, Robinson AHN, LeCoultre B, et al. Patellar tendon length: the factor in patellar instability? Knee 2002;9:3–6.

[116] Simmons E Jr, Cameron JC. Patella alta and recurrent dislocation of the patella. Clin Orthop 1992;274:265–9.

[117] Andrish JT. The elmslie-trillat procedure. Tech Orthop 1997;12:1–8.

[118] Kumar A, Jones S, Bickerstaff DR, et al. Functional evaluation of the modified elmslie–trillat procedure for patello-femoral dysfunction. Knee 2001;8:287–92.

[119] Fulkerson JP, Becker GJ, Meaney JA, et al. Anteromedial tibial tubercle transfer without bone graft. Am J Sports Med 1990;18:490–7.

[120] Nomura E, Inoue M. Cartilage lesions of the patella in recurrent patellar dislocation. Am J Sports Med 2004;32:498–502.

[121] Post WR. Open patellar realignment for patellar pain and instability. Oper Tech Sports Med 1994;2:297–302.

[122] Peterson L, Karlsson J, Brittberg M. Patellar instability with recurrent dislocation due to patellofemoral dysplasia results after surgical treatment. Bull Hosp Jt Dis Orthop Inst 1988;48:130–9.

[123] Slocum B, Slocum TD. Trochlear wedge recession for medial patellar luxation. Vet Clin North Am Small Anim Pract 1993;23:869–75.

[124] Kuroda R, Kambic H, Valdevit A, et al. Distribution of patellofemoral joint pressures after femoral trochlear osteotomy. Knee Surg Sports Traumatol Arthrosc 2002;10:33–7.

[125] Albee FH. The bone graft wedge in the treatment of habitual dislocation of the patella. Medical Record 1915;88:257–9.

[126] Weiker GT, Black KP. The anterior femoral osteotomy for patellofemoral instability. Am J Knee Surg 1997;10:221–7.

[127] Masse Y. Trochleoplasty: restoration of the intercondylar groove in subluxations and dislocations of the patella. Rev Chir Orthop Reparatrice Appar Mot 1978;64:3–17.

[128] Haspl M, Cicak N, Klobucar H, et al. Fully arthroscopic stabilization of the patella. Arthroscopy 2002;18:1–3.

[129] Small NC, Glogau AI, Berezin MA. Arthroscopically assisted proximal extensor mechanism realignment of the knee. Arthroscopy 1993;9:63–7, American Academy of Orthopaedic Surgeons.

Autologous Chondrocyte Implantation and Anteromedialization in the Treatment of Patellofemoral Chondrosis

Jack Farr, II, MD[a,b,*]

[a]OrthoIndy Knee Care Institute, 5255 E Stop 11 Road, Suite 300, Indianapolis, IN 46237, USA
[b]Indiana University School of Medicine, Department of Orthopaedic Surgery, 541 Clinical Drive, Suite 600, Indianapolis, IN 46202, USA

Treatment of patellofemoral (PF) chondrosis continues to evolve. While articular cartilage is aneural, damage and loss of articular cartilage is often associated with pain in the affected joint or joint compartment, such as the PF compartment. The association is indirect, as the pain originates from subchondral bone or soft tissues; thus, allocating pain to chondrosis is by exclusion of the myriad of other causes of PF pain. During this "diagnosis by exclusion," the mosaic of other PF pain causes must be appreciated and treated concomitantly with any chondrosis treatment. PF chondrosis is often associated with abnormal PF stress such as lateral compression or excessive lateral position of the patella in the trochlea. Anteromedialization (AMZ), a treatment for such abnormalities, was popularized by Fulkerson [1]. Review of AMZ outcomes by Pidoriano and colleagues [2] revealed poor outcomes with advanced chondrosis in certain PF regions. In the same era, Brittberg and colleagues [3] reported that cartilage restoration of PF chondrosis with autologous chondrocyte implantation (ACI) had poor outcomes when PF malalignment (excessive lateral patellar position) was not corrected. Subsequently, several authors have shown that by combining AMZ and ACI, very positive outcomes are possible [4–8].

Anteromedialization

Tibial tuberosity surgery has a long history, which was initially developed empirically. Medialization of the tuberosity was designed to decrease an abnormal quadriceps angle (Q angle) and redirect an excessively lateral patella to a more normal central position in the trochlea. Maquet [9] used two-dimensional mechanical calculations to predict that the force vectors acting at the patellofemoral compartment would decrease with tibial tuberosity anterization. Fulkerson [1] combined these approaches with an inclined osteotomy that allowed components of anterization and medialization (hence anteromedialization). Fulkerson's initial series success in 1983 was reinforced by the durability of long-term outcomes of AMZ as reported by Buuck and Fulkerson [10]. The original technique of Fulkerson is well described in his book, *Disorders of the Patellofemoral Joint*, and was later modified by Farr using a commercially available jig [11,12]. This is briefly described in the technique below ("AMZ with ACI Operative Technique").

Before focusing on the surgical technique, it is important to emphasize that patients considered for AMZ should have failed a thorough physical therapy program with emphasis on proximal musculature and core muscle strengthening. The pain should be activity related and have no component of complex regional pain syndrome, malingering, or secondary gain. The pain should be focused at the patellofemoral joint and associated with symptomatic lateral tilt and/or excessive

* OrthoIndy Knee Care Institute, 5255 E Stop 11 Road Suite 300, Indianapolis, IN 46237.
E-mail address: jfarr@orthindy.com

lateral position of the patella (chronic patellar status subluxation) and an increased tibial tuberosity-trochlear groove distance (TT-TG), which may be assessed by CT or MRI [13]. In addition, full appreciation of the underlying alterations of PF biomechanics is important. Cohen and colleagues [14] showed the variable decreases in PF stress with AMZ using finite element analysis that averages approximately 20% rather than the calculated 50% of Maquet [9]. The cadaver study of Kuroda and colleagues highlighted the undesirable medial knee overload with overly zealous medialization; this further emphasizes the importance of preoperative measurement of the TT-TG distances to aid in planning the extent of medialization [15]. The TT-TG distance associated with recurrent lateral patellar instability is over 15 to 20 mm, while the mean of asymptomatic patients has been reported as 13 [13]. The end goal of medialization is to reposition the tuberosity to achieve a TT-TG distance of approximately less than 15 mm, certainly avoiding low single digits as per Kuroda and Andrish. The optimal extent of elevation remains under debate. The literature recommends a range of elevation between 10 and 15 mm (for details of these results please refer to an annotated table of anterization studies by Schepsis and Watson [16]). With the goal of 10 to 15 mm of anterization, the extent of medialization desired can be calculated preoperatively using simple trigonometry. For example, the steepest slope possible for AMZ is approximately 60 degrees. Using the triangle rule, 15 mm of anterization with this slope will yield a medialization of 8.7 mm. With a constant amount of elevation, the medialization may be increased by decreasing the slope (eg, 45 degree slope = 15 mm anterization and 15 mm of medialization). If the patient has excessive lateral tilt, lateral step cut lengthening or titrated lateral release can be performed concomitantly. If the patient has patholaxity of the medial patellofemoral ligament, repair or reconstruction of the ligament may be performed concomitantly with AMZ. The goal is to optimize the biomechanical environment of the PF compartment for cartilage restoration.

As this paper is specifically discussing AMZ with autologous cultured chondroctye implantation or ACI (in the United States the product is distributed under the name Carticel by Genzyme, Cambridge, MA), additional levels of decision making are involved. As ACI is a two-staged procedure (stage one: arthroscopic harvest of a cartilage biopsy, stage two: implantation), the AMZ can be performed at the time of the arthroscopy and biopsy or at the time of implantation. Several factors affect this decision. First, in isolation, both AMZ and ACI are moderately large procedures with recoveries requiring weeks to months. Both result in dehabilitation and the need for extensive rehabilitation. These first two considerations would suggest performing the arthroscopic biopsy alone and the AMZ at the time of ACI. By combining the procedures, the exposure for the ACI is straightforward; however, insurance medical policies introduce complications. Preauthorization for ACI at the patellofemoral compartment sometimes requires several months to obtain. The difficulty of preauthorization is a result of Food and Drug Administration (FDA)-approved indications (only for articular cartilage defects of the trochlea and medial and lateral femoral condyles). As patellar and bipolar (patellofemoral) chondral defects are not included in these indications ("off label"), proof of efficacy and safety must be presented to the insurance companies to validate the use of ACI in these situations (peer-reviewed literature is often used as documentation for this). Even after documentation is submitted to insurance companies, some preauthorizations require months to years. In these situations, AMZ may be considered a first step, assuming the articular cartilage lesions are located in regions that are expected to have satisfactory results. (According to Pidoriano' and colleagues study, optimal results were noted in patients with distal lateral patellar chondrosis and intact trochlear cartilage. Poor results after AMZ were noted in knees with proximal pole chondrosis, medial patellar chondrosis, panpatellar chondrosis, and when the trochlea was involved [2].) These areas of chondrosis that do poorly with an isolated AMZ are the basis for combining AMZ with cartilage restoration. On the other hand, if preauthorization for PF ACI is expected, combining AMZ and ACI would allow for one time off of school or work, one rehabilitation, and one major knee surgery.

Assuming preauthorization is achieved, the plans should be reviewed with the patient. By following the technique details, a good surgical outcome is possible. However, a good "surgical outcome" in the face of a patient with persistent pain is, in fact, a failure. As such, proper patient selection and preoperative expectation counseling is extremely important. Many patients have unrealistic expectations and these need to be modified preoperatively. The surgeon physician's goal is to decrease pain and improve function, while the patient's "preexpectation counseling" goal is often no pain with all desired activities. Once again, patellofemoral pain is a complex mosaic as eloquently detailed by Dye [17]. As considerable time may have passed from the first decision to proceed with AMZ/ACI, thorough reassessment of the patient is important to be sure all other aspects of PF pain have been addressed and preoperative rehabilitation has been optimized. While obtaining informed consent from the patient, the expected postoperative course and time to achieve specific activity goals should be reviewed.

AMZ with ACI operative technique

In the setting of ACI concomitant with AMZ, a longitudinal incision courses from the level of the quadriceps tendon to 10 cm distal to the patellar tendon attachment to the tibial tuberosity. The subcutaneous tissues are elevated to expose the lateral capsule, the patellar tendon, tibial tuberosity, and the anterior musculature compartment (Fig. 1). In light of the pathology that has led to the choice of AMZ, most of these knees have an excessively tight lateral retinaculum. Therefore, the most common deep approach is lateral, which also avoids insult to the medial quadriceps. As it is optimal to seal the joint after ACI, an option to lateral release is a step cut lateral lengthening. At the 2006 International Patellofemoral Study Group meeting, Biedert described the step cut lengthening. To perform the step cut lengthening, the superficial layer that is confluent with the expansion from the iliotibial band is incised and elevated posteriorly for 2 cm. An incision is then made through the lateral

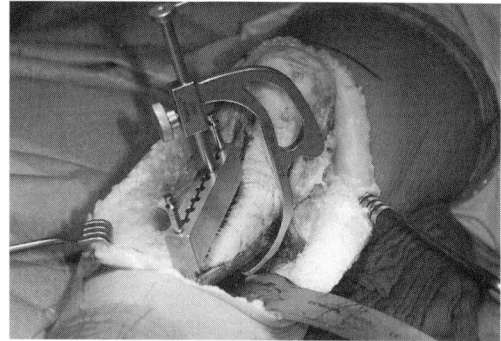

Fig. 2. Slope selector predicts osteotomy exit.

patellofemoral ligaments, capsule, and synovium 2 cm posterior to the previous incision. This allows for up to 2 cm of lateral lengthening.

The deep incision is carried distally past the patellar tendon along the lateral aspect of the tibial tuberosity. At the proximal extent of the anterior compartment, an incision is made just distal of the insertion of the iliotibial band on Gerdy's tubercle. The anterior compartment musculature is bluntly elevated from the lateral face of the tibia to the posterior border. A blunt custom retractor is placed subperiosteally both to retract the anterior compartment and to protect the deep neurovascular structures. To allow elevation without abnormal forces in the medial soft tissues, an incision is made medially immediately adjacent to the patellar tendon. An Army-Navy retractor isolates and protects the patellar tendon.

A custom cutting block (Tracker AMZ set, DePuy Mitek, Raynum, NJ) is positioned on the tibial tuberosity (Fig. 2). Proximally, the jig is immediately medial to the patellar tendon insertion on the tibial tuberosity while distally it courses

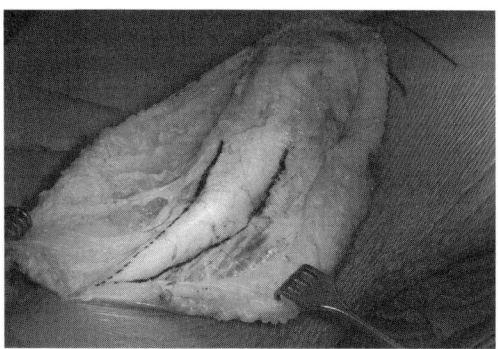

Fig. 1. Tuberosity position is excessively lateral as per MRI.

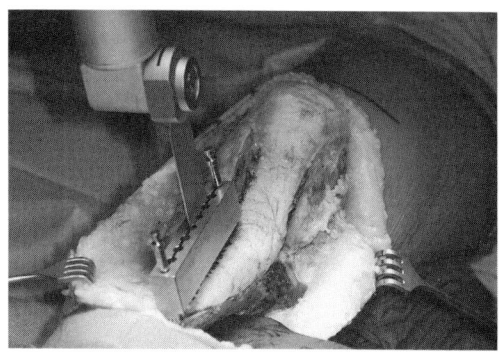

Fig. 3. Saw cut through secured cutting block jig.

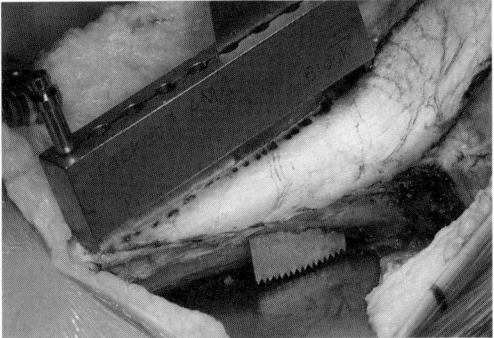

Fig. 4. Custom retractor protects neurovascular structures.

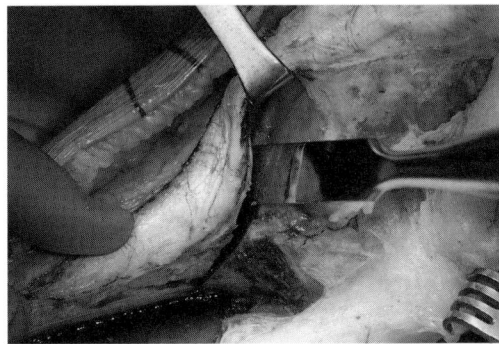

Fig. 6. Second proximal cut: proximal to patellar tendon.

laterally to allow the osteotomy to exit on the lateral wall of the tibial. The slope has been planned preoperatively to determine the extent of medialization with a constant elevation of between 10 and 15 mm. The slope is then set with the slope selector arm temporarily attached to the cutting block with the arm tip showing the exit of the osteotomy (see Fig. 2). The osteotomy for the maximum slope of 60 degrees exits just anterior to the posterior wall of the tibia. Decreasing the slope increases the medialization for the same elevation with the other reproducible angle of 45 degrees yielding the same excursion medially as anteriorly.

After confirming the position of the cutting block to affect the desired slope, the cutting block is temporarily fixed with two pins. An oscillating saw cooled with saline makes the cut through the captured cutting block and is observed to exit posteriorly along the lateral wall of the tibial with the retractor protecting deep tissues (Figs. 3 and 4). The cutting block is removed. The proximal and distal cuts of the sloped osteotomy are completed with the oscillating saw using the first cut in the same manner as a captured guide. To complete the osteotomy, osteotomes are used first to connect to proximal posterior cut to the lateral attachment site of the patellar tendon to the tibial tuberosity (Fig. 5). The final cut is made just proximal to the patellar tendon attachment to the tibial tuberosity lateral to medial while the patellar tendon is protected with an Army-Navy retractor (Fig. 6). The tuberosity is now free and may be retracted during the cartilage defect preparation, patch templating, and cell implantation under the sealed patch (Figs. 7–11). After the ACI is completed, the tuberosity is held in an anteromedial position (Fig. 12) and fixed with two 4.5 mm interfragmentary screws followed by measuring the extent of anterization and medialization (Fig. 13A,B; Fig. 14). Optionally, after the AMZ is fixed, the medial patellofemoral ligament can then be tightened or reconstructed (Figs. 15 and 16).

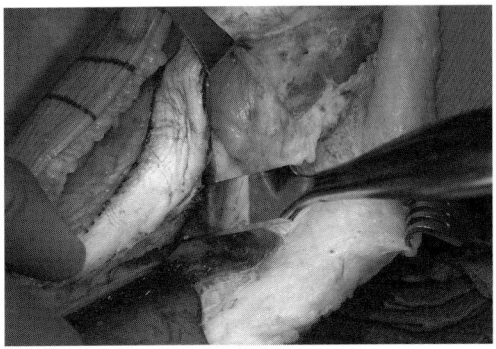

Fig. 5. First proximal cut: posterior to patellar tendon.

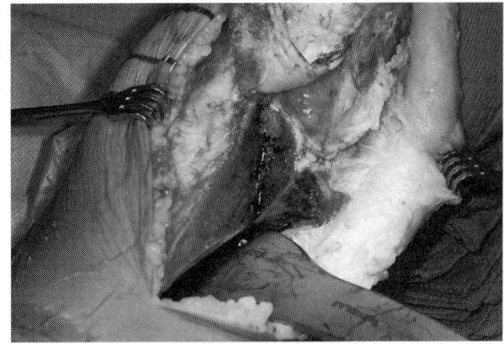

Fig. 7. Steep slope of osteotomy.

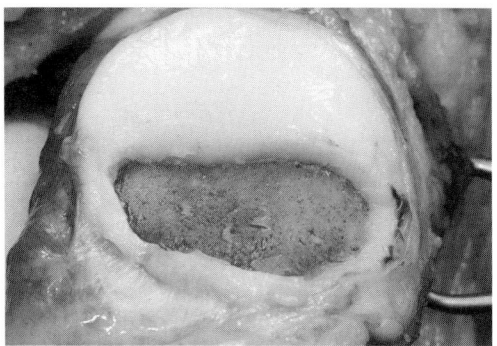

Fig. 8. Patellar chondral defect debrided to subchondral bone.

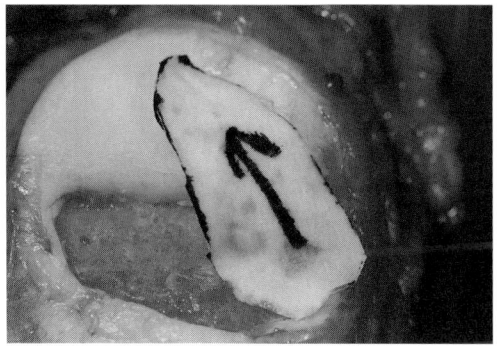

Fig. 9. Periosteal patch sized to fit defect.

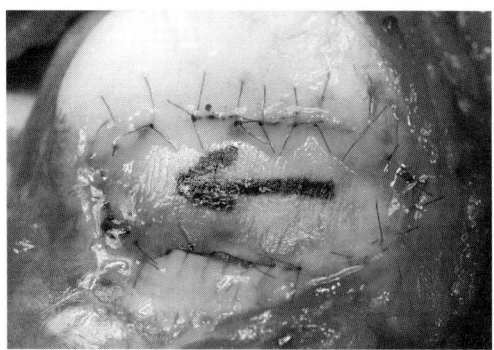

Fig. 10. Suture and sealed patch after chondrocyte implantation.

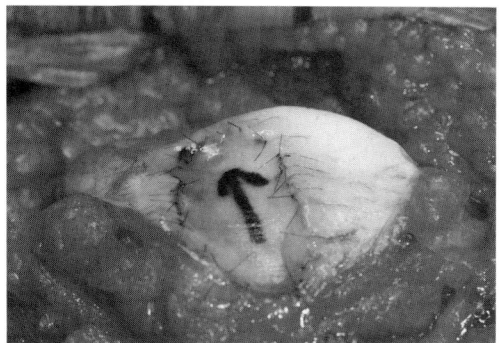

Fig. 11. Patch follows articular cartilage topology.

Results and discussion of AMZ and ACI

In 2002, Peterson reported marked improvements with PF ACI outcomes compared with the 1994 paper of Brittberg and colleagues [3,4]. With the addition of AMZ, Peterson and colleagues reported 11 of 17 PF ACI patients with good and excellent results at 2 years and 13 of 17 at 2 to 9 years [18]. Minas and Bryant [5] confirmed these findings in 2005 with 71% good or excellent results in 45 patients noting that 62% of the PF ACI patients received AMZ. Henderson and Lavigne [6] reported similar results for PF ACI yet he divided his patients into two groups. Those with clinically perceived malalignment underwent AMZ with PF ACI and those with clinically normal alignment only receiving PF ACI. The group with AMZ PF ACI had 86% good and excellent outcomes, while the isolated PF ACI patients had 54% good and excellent results yielding a combined 71% good and excellent outcomes. Henderson suggested that slight unappreciated malalignments might have led to the lower response in those patients without concomitant

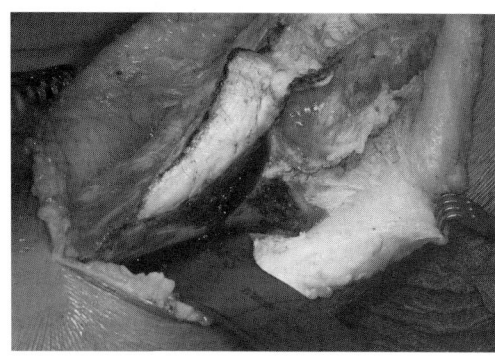

Fig. 12. Tuberosity pedicle moved anteromedially.

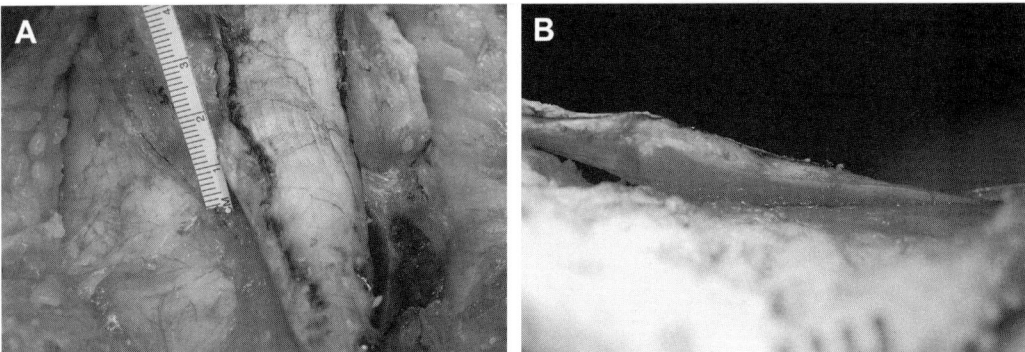

Fig. 13. (*A*) After fixation, 12 mm of anterization. (*B*) After fixation, 12 mm of anterization.

AMZ (note that the TT-TG distance was not measured). Additionally, the role of AMZ in lowering PF stress is not fully understood, as Steinwach and Kreuz [7] reported overall 87% good and excellent results in 10 trochlear ACI and 19 patellar ACI patients noting that none had an AMZ as all had reported normal alignment. We reported 80% (31 of 39) good and excellent PF ACI outcomes in patients followed for more than 2 years [8]. Within this group, like Henderson, we clinically assessed PF alignment and only performed AMZ with PF ACI on those perceived to have malalignment. Twenty-eight patients had concomitant AMZ and ACI. We reported no significant difference between those with and without AMZ, nor were there differences between monopolar and bipolar lesions. To investigate the possible role of ACI in improving isolated AMZ results, the AMZ outcomes of various PF chondrosis patterns is a baseline. Pidoriano and colleagues reported the following outcomes of isolated AMZ patients: 56% of patients with medial facet patellar lesions (Type III) had good results and 20% of patients with proximal pole or panpatellar lesions (Type IV) had good outcomes. Patients with central trochlear lesions had largely poor results with anteromedial AMZ. In our PF ACI group, all treated patellar lesions were Type III or IV, and 56% of trochlear lesions were located in the central region of the trochlea. Those treated with ACI and AMZ had 75% (21 of 28) of patients with a good to excellent result. These improvements compared with AMZ alone support the earlier studies of Peterson and colleagues [4], Minas and Bryant [5], and Henderson and Lavigne [6].

These case series support the safety and efficacy of PF ACI in the short and intermediate term. The role of AMZ appears to be important in those patients with malalignment, but the clinical experience of the surgeons is difficult to objectively communicate based on the available data. It may be useful, in the future, to evaluate patients pre- and postoperatively for PF contact areas similar to the FEA modeling of Ateshian and Cohen, as well as

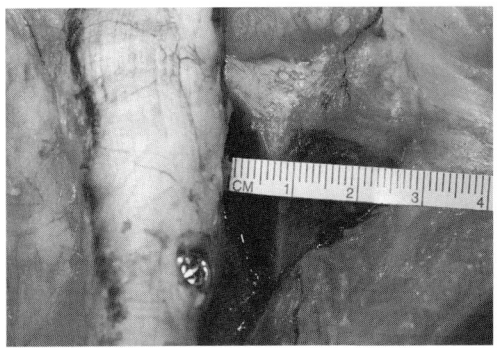

Fig. 14. After fixation, 6 mm of medialization.

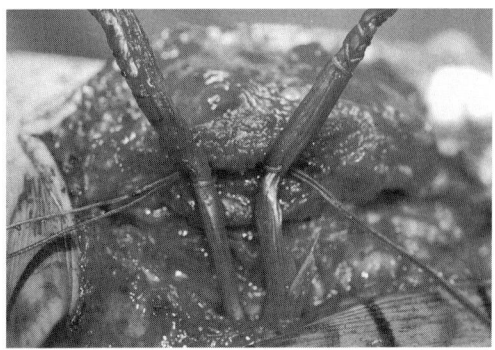

Fig. 15. After AMZ, MPFL reconstruction lengths set.

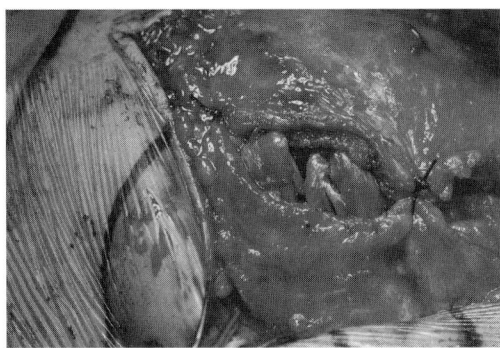

Fig. 16. MPFL grafts folded back in preparation for suturing.

measurement of the TT-TG distance and then correlate these with outcomes in an effort to further add objectively [13,14,19]. Hopefully, by using objective data points preoperatively, the optimal use of AMZ with ACI may be elucidated.

References

[1] Fulkerson JP. Anteromedialization of the tibial tuberosity for patellofemoral malalignment. Clin Orthop Relat Res 1983;177:176–81.

[2] Pidoriano AJ, Weinstein RN, Buuck DA, et al. Correlation of patellar articular lesions with results from anteromedial tibial tubercle transfer. Am J Sports Med 1997;25:533–7.

[3] Brittberg M, Lindahl A, Nilsson A, et al. Treatment of deep cartilage defects in the knee with autologous chondrocyte transplantation. N Engl J Med 1994; 331:889–95.

[4] Peterson L, Brittberg M, Kiviranta I, et al. Autologous chondrocyte transplantation biomechanics and long-term durability. Am J Sports Med 2002;30:2–12.

[5] Minas T, Bryant T. The role of autologous chondrocyte implantation in the patellofemoral joint. Clin Orthop Relat Res 2005;436:30–9.

[6] Henderson IP, Lavigne P. Periosteal autologous chondrocyte implantation for patellar chondral defect in patients with normal and abnormal patellar tracking. Knee 2006;13:274–9.

[7] Steinwachs M, Kreuz PC. Autologous chondrocyte implantation in chondral defects of the knee with a type I/III collagen membrane: a prospective study with a 3-year follow-up. Arthroscopy 2007;23:381–7.

[8] Farr J. Autologous chondrocyte implantation improves patellofemoral cartilage treatment outcomes. Clin Orthop and Rel Res 2007;463:187–94.

[9] Maquet P. Biomecanique de l'articulation patellofemoral. Acta Orthop Belg 1978;44:41–54.

[10] Buuck D, Fulkerson J. Anteromedialization of the tibial tubercle: a 4–12 year follow up. Oper Tech Sports Med 2000;8:131–7.

[11] Fulkerson JP. Surgical treatment of patellofemoral chondrosis and arthrosis. In: Cook DB, Klaus FM, editors. Disorders of the patellofemoral joint. 3rd edition. Baltimore (MD): Williams and Wilkins; 1997. p. 299–336.

[12] Farr J. Anteromedialization of the tibial tubercle for treatment of patellofemoral malpositioning and concomitant isolated patellofemoral arthrosis. Tech Orthop 1997;12:151–64.

[13] Schoettle PB, Zanetti M, Seifert B, et al. The tibial tuberosity-trochlear groove distance: a comparative study between CT and MRI scanning. The Knee 2006;13:26–31.

[14] Cohen ZA, Henry JH, McCarthy DM, et al. Computer simulations of patellofemoral joint surgery. Patient-specific models for tuberosity transfer. Am J Sports Med 2003;31(1):87–98.

[15] Kuroda R, Kambic H, Valdevit A, et al. Articular cartilage contact pressure after tibial tuberosity transfer. Am J Sports Med 2001;29(4):403–9.

[16] Schepsis AA, Watson JF. Patellofemoral arthritis with malalignment. In: Fulkerson JP, editor. Monograph series 29: common patellofemoral problems. Rosemont (IL): American Academy of Orthopaedic Surgeons; 2005. p. 57–71.

[17] Dye SF. The pathophysiology of patellofemoral pain: a tissue homeostasis perspective. Clin Orthop and Rel Res 2005;436:100–10.

[18] Peterson L, Minas T, Brittberg M, et al. Two- to 9-year outcome after autologous chondrocyte transplantation of the knee. Clin Orthop Relat Res 2000;374:212–34.

[19] Ateshian GA, Hung CT. Patellofemoral joint biomechanics and tissue engineering. Clin Orthop and Rel Res 2005;81:81–90.

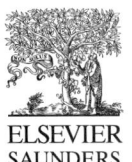

Focal Anatomic Patellofemoral Inlay Resurfacing: Theoretic Basis, Surgical Technique, and Case Reports

Philip A. Davidson, MD[a,b,*], Dennis Rivenburgh, MS, ATC, PA-C[b]

[a]Department of Orthopaedic Surgery, University of South Florida, 6500 66th St. N, Pinellas Park, FL 33781, USA
[b]Tampa Bay Orthopaedic Specialists, Pinellas Park, FL 33781, USA

Isolated patellofemoral degenerative changes range from 11% in men to 24% in women over the age of 55 years with symptomatic osteoarthritis of the knee [1]. Reports show an incidence of isolated patellofemoral arthritis in 9.2% of patients over 40 years [2]. The review of patients undergoing patellofemoral arthroplasty shows that the majority are women [3–8]. This may well be attributed to a higher incidence of congenital malalignment and dysplasia in women [9]. In their study of 31,516 knee arthroscopies, Curl and colleagues [10] reported approximately 20% of cases with patellar articular defects and 15% with trochlear articular pathology. Although these findings may have variable clinical significance at the time of index arthroscopy, the biomechanical alteration of the articulation may indicate a tendency for progressive degeneration. Anterior knee pain associated with patellofemoral degeneration is a very common presenting complaint to musculoskeletal health care providers, especially in active or elderly women.

A multitude of factors guide treatment of patellofemoral pathology, including patient age, presenting symptoms, body type, articular morphology, static and dynamic alignment, and imaging studies. When conservative measures fail, the most common surgical procedures include debridement, chondroplasty, soft tissue or bony realignment, biologic cartilage restoration, patellectomy, total knee arthroplasty, and patellofemoral arthroplasty [8,11–18].

In patients with normal patellar alignment and traumatic localized defects, standard biologic treatment options have been the mainstay of first-round surgical interventions. Biologic resurfacing described for the patellofemoral joint includes marrow stimulation techniques or biologic reconstruction. Marrow stimulation techniques include microfracture, abrasion, picking, and drilling. Biologic restoration methods include osteochondral autografts, osteochondral allografts, chondrocyte implantation, and scaffold resurfacing. Results from the biologic spectrum of treatment options have been reported with variable success rates [19–22]. Patients with chronic malalignment or dysplasia typically show degenerative, rather than focal, patellofemoral articular disease. These patients often require concomitant soft tissue and bony procedures to address the entire realm of pathologies related to the extensor mechanism and anterior knee.

Prosthetic patellofemoral inlay resurfacing is a novel treatment concept introduced to the orthopedic community in 2006. The theoretic basis of this type of arthroplasty entails recreating ambient anatomy based on intraoperative topographic mapping. The implant is intrinsically stable by virtue of the inset position relative to the surrounding joint surface. Furthermore, using this strategy, concurrent soft tissue and bony surgery is facilitated, because volume is not extrinsically added to the joint. This type of surgery, in contradistinction to some procedures labeled as "minimally invasive" is in fact "microinvasive." This is accomplished with smaller exposures, shorter operating times, simple and cannulated implantation technique, minimal bone resection, and typically less peri-operative blood loss. Resurfacing, per se, has been widely accepted for shoulder and hip

* Corresponding author. Department of Orthopaedic Surgery, University of South Florida, 6500 66th St. N, Pinellas Park, FL 33781.
E-mail address: pdavidson@tampabayortho.com (P.A. Davidson).

indications with typically near-complete unipolar articular coverage. The HemiCAP resurfacing platform technology (Arthrosurface, Inc. Franklin, MA, USA) reflects a new paradigm in joint resurfacing, based on intraoperative joint surface mapping, making use of a corresponding patient-specific implant. This system allows for restoration of complex geometric surfaces in a variety of morphologic and pathologic states. Various diameter sizes are available across a multitude of joints, using the same platform technologic principles [23–28]. The current patellofemoral HemiCAP resurfacing prosthesis is available in 20-mm diameter and focuses on relatively localized defects of the distal trochlear surface and patellar defects. The prosthesis incorporates a trochlear articular component that is connected to a fixation stud via a taper interlock and a modular polyethylene patella component (Fig. 1). A choice of 13 different offset dimensions allows for a patient-specific geometry match in the distal trochlear. Larger diameter implants are pending, to address more diffuse patellofemoral disease.

Patient assessment

It is important to determine the source of anterior knee pain. Physical examination includes assessment of the kinematic chain during normal gait and deep knee flexion from hip to ankle. Particular attention is directed to patellar alignment with signs of tilt and subluxation. In addition, the examination assesses the medial and lateral facets, articular crepitus, particular local pain foci, and quadriceps strength.

Patients suffering from patellofemoral disease typically exhibit anterior knee pain with the extensor mechanism under load. Weight-bearing radiographs allow for improved patellofemoral assessment and include standard anteroposterior, notch view at 30° of flexion, lateral, and an axial weight-bearing Merchant view at 45° of knee flexion [23]. Chondral damage, soft tissues including patellar and quadriceps tendons, and patellofemoral joint symmetry or dysplasia can be assessed further and quantified on magnetic resonance imaging.

Focal patellofemoral resurfacing alone cannot be effective in global degenerative joint disease. Therefore, relatively monocompartmental pathology has to be verified. Patellofemoral pathology must be confirmed at the time of surgery to consider patients for patellofemoral resurfacing.

Indications and contraindications

The HemiCAP patellofemoral resurfacing prosthesis is intended for patients with pain and functional limitations who have not responded to conservative treatment measures or previous surgical procedures and have cartilage defects or degeneration limited to the patellofemoral joint. Both medial and lateral tibiofemoral compartments should be substantially normal or surgically addressed to render them such. Patients should show normal patellofemoral alignment, or as an alternative, improved patellar tracking can be addressed intraoperatively with concurrent procedures. Normal joint stability, both tibiofemoral and patellofemoral, and relatively good range of motion should be demonstrated before surgery.

Contraindications include diffuse full-thickness articular cartilage loss extending beyond the implant, extensive bone loss, infection, advanced osteoporosis, and other metabolic or inflammatory disorders that may negatively affect implant fixation or render the joint prone to continued degeneration.

Surgical technique

Patellofemoral HemiCAP implantation is performed with a combination of arthroscopic and

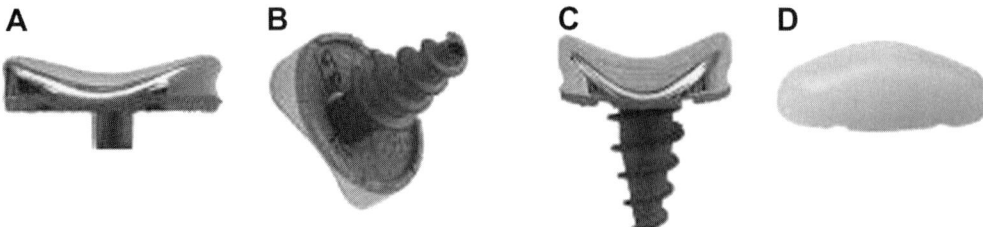

Fig. 1. (*A*) Trochlear resurfacing component (example with shallow trochlear offsets): cobalt-chromium alloy (Co-Cr-Mo). (*B*) Trochlear component. Undersurface coating: titanium (CP Ti); fixation stud: titanium alloy (Ti-6Al-4V). (*C*) Trochlear component (example with deep offsets) and connected fixation stud. (*D*) Patellar component (example with anatomic ridge): ultra-high-molecular weight polyethylene (UHMWPE).

open surgery. The patient is positioned in the supine position, standard arthroscopic portals are placed, and the joint is inspected. Arthroscopic treatment is performed for concurrent pathologies and to confirm proper indication for prosthetic implantation. At the conclusion of the arthroscopic procedure, an arthroscopic lateral release may be performed. This may be indicated for patellofemoral realignment purposes and may also be used to facilitate exposure subsequently. The procedure is now converted into an open surgery by extending the medial portal between 4 and 7 cm, depending on the size of the patient. Alternatively a midline incision may be used. Electrocautery is used to incise the medial capsule and patellofemoral retinaculum with care to prevent damage to the underlying articular cartilage. The capsular incision can be extended either proximally or distally, depending on the patient morphology. A soft tissue sleeve of approximately 1 cm is left attached to the patella for subsequent closure and medial plication, if necessary. Bony realignment, when indicated, can be performed at this point in the procedure. The medial tissues are tagged and reflected, and the patella can be inverted to either 90° or 180°, depending on surgeon preference. A retractor is placed over the lateral condyle, reflecting the patella in the lateral direction, providing access to the trochlear groove.

With the knee in 90° of flexion, the HemiCAP drill guide is seated with four points of contact. The footed guide is placed in an anterior position to develop a working axis normal to the distal trochlear articular surface (Fig. 2).

The fully cannulated instrumentation initiates prosthetic alignment by placing a guide pin into the center of the trochlear defect. A step drill is advanced over the guide pin until the proximal shoulder is flush to the articular surface. Care is taken to avoid overdrilling, so as not to compromise subsequent screw fixation in subchondral bone. Standard tapping technique is used before the fixation screw is placed into the center of the defect. Etched depth markings provide external reference points while advancing instruments to ultimately achieve flush prosthetic implantation. Once peak height placement of the fixation screw is verified with a trial cap, a centering shaft is seated into the taper head of the fixation component to enable its navigational properties.

A contact probe is placed over the centering shaft and rotated to obtain superior/inferior and medial/lateral offsets (Fig. 3). A corresponding reamer prepares the implant bed (Fig. 4). A sizing trial with matching offsets is used to confirm a congruent fit of the trochlear component to the edge of the surrounding articular surface. Before placement of the final trochlear component, the procedure is directed toward preparation of the patellar implant.

The patella's anterior-to-posterior thickness is verified to accommodate the patella component with a reaming depth of typically 6.5 mm. With the knee at 90° flexion, an alignment guide facilitates target placement of the patella component while observing range of motion. A guide pin is placed into the previously identified location—a drill guide again provides placement

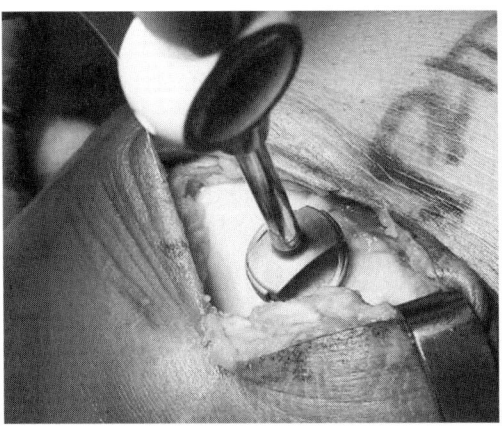

Fig. 2. Drill guide placement in the center of the trochlear defect, perpendicular to the joint surface.

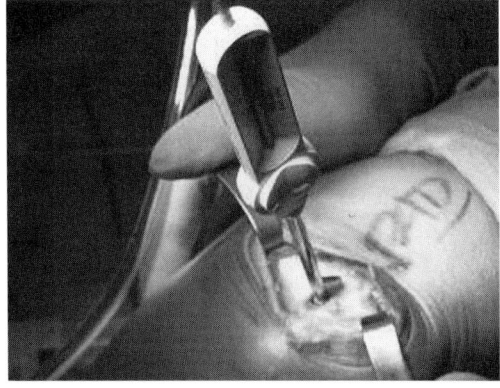

Fig. 3. Contact probe inserted over centering shaft, which is placed in the fixation component.

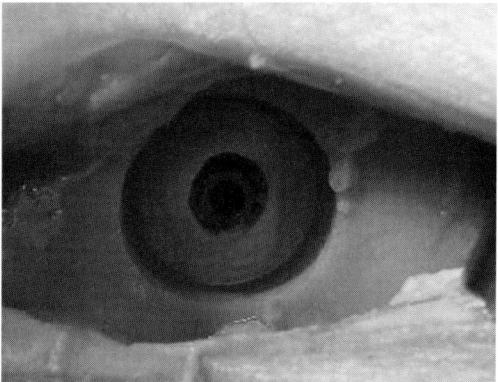

Fig. 4. Final trochlear implant bed after high-speed reaming.

within a normal working axis to the patellar surface (Fig. 5).

A cannulated drill is advanced over the guide pin until the distal shoulder of the drill is flush to the articular surface. Using a powered drill, the patella centering shaft is placed over the guide pin until it reaches the distal laser marked depth marking. The contact probe establishes patellar offsets in two dimensions. A corresponding reamer is preparing the implant bed in the patella, and a sizing trial allows verification of congruent margin fit to the surrounding articular surface (Fig. 6A and B).

An anatomic or flat patellar contour can be trialed to ensure optimized tracking. The final patellar component is aligned on the implant holder and cemented into the prepared socket (Fig. 6C). The femoral trochlear component is now aligned with the appropriate offsets on the implant holder and placed into the taper of the fixation screw (Fig. 7).

A mallet and impactor firmly seat the trochlear component. Once implantation is complete, a trial range of motion is performed. A stable and balanced extensor mechanism should be present or achieved with concurrent procedures.

Closure of the medial retinacular incision is performed using standard capsular sutures. If a proximal realignment is necessary, the medial capsule can be plicated during the capsular closure. The lateral retinacular incision is left open.

Case reports

Case 1

A 45-year-old woman, an athletically active physical education teacher, presented with bilateral knee pain for more than 20 years not associated with any trauma or patellar dislocations. Both knees had two previous knee arthroscopic debridements and no realignment procedures. None of those surgeries gave sustained relief. At the time of presentation, the patient stated "I cannot do anything because of my knees; I am extremely limited in what I can do. I can't get up and down from a chair without difficulties, I can't do athletic maneuvers, and doing my job is nearly impossible. I have a constant sensation of aching made worse with any activities, and it clearly feels like there's bone on bone."

Preoperative physical examination showed symmetric findings bilaterally. Range of motion was 0° to 140°. There was painful arc of motion with palpable and audible crepitance from 40° to 140°. Marked pain was noted with patellofemoral compression. The Q angle was 9°, and the patient had symmetric quad atrophy compared with other lower extremity muscle groups. The knee was stable, and she had no specific pain with patellar lateral apprehension testing. The medial and lateral compartments were unremarkable, and the knee was stable with a small effusion. Preoperative radiographs showed advanced isolated patellofemoral arthrosis with lateral patellar subluxation.

Index procedure

The patient underwent left knee diagnostic arthroscopy to confirm the appropriate indications. Intraoperative findings included a 50% full-thickness loss of articular cartilage in the distal

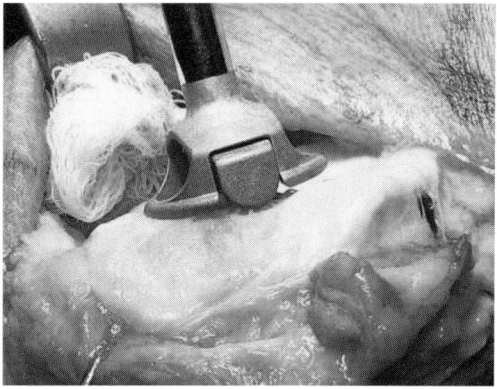

Fig. 5. Patellar drill guide placement in the center of the defect.

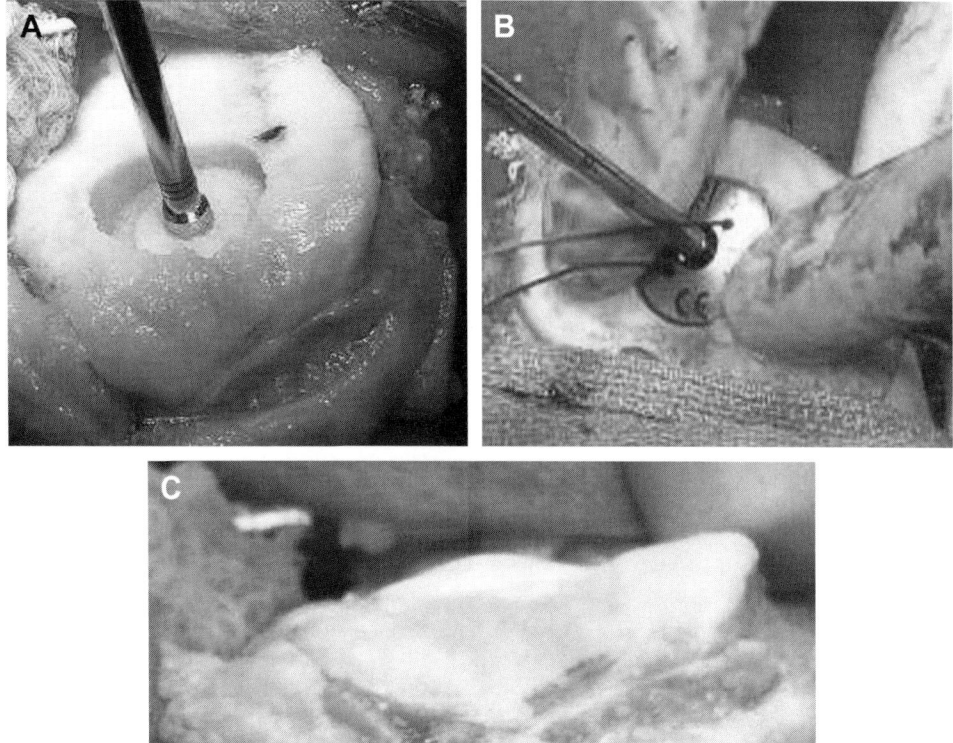

Fig. 6. (*A*) Preparation of patellar implant bed. (*B*) Sizing trial to verify congruent articular margins. (*C*) Final patellar component implanted.

trochlear. The patella had loss of cartilage on the lateral facet and the patellar ridge. The medial and lateral compartments were without pathologic change.

A mini-open patellofemoral resurfacing with the bipolar Arthrosurface HemiCAP device and an arthroscopic lateral release were performed. During closure, a proximal realignment with medial retinacular plication was performed. The surgery was done as an outpatient procedure with minimal blood loss. The patient had range of motion from 0° to 65° by the first postoperative week and 105° by the third postoperative week, and she returned to work with a cane by the fourth postoperative week. She regained 140° flexion by the eighth postoperative week. Rehabilitation included immediate full weight-bearing, no imposed limitation of flexion, and use of axillary crutches for 4 weeks. After her experience with this procedure, 10 months after the first patellofemoral resurfacing, she elected to have the contralateral knee treated with a similar procedure. Her second knee underwent a nearly identical operation with similar results. At last follow-up, the patient expressed a high degree of satisfaction for both knees (Table 1). Please note that at the time of surgery, excellent articular congruity was achieved for the trochlear component. Fig. 8B shows an apparent offset relative to the subchondral bone, but this implant had circumferential congruity with the ambient surface (Figs. 7–11).

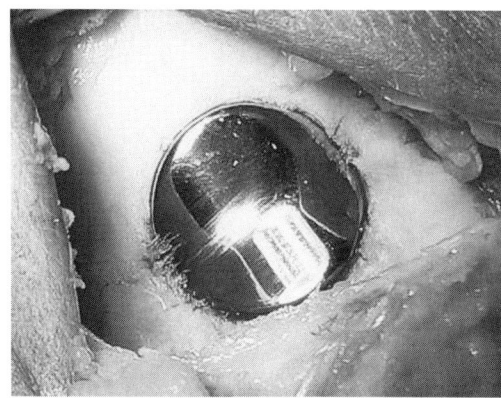

Fig. 7. Final trochlear component implanted.

Table 1
Case 1: outcomes measures for left knee with 12 months of follow-up and right knee with 3 months of follow-up

Outcomes score		Preoperative assessment	Last follow-up assessment	Percent improvement
SF-36 (Physical)	L	32.4	51.2	58
	R	34.3	44.1	20.7
IKDC	L	26.2	75	186.4
	R	33/4	57.2	70.1
Fulkerson knee score	L	57	96	68.4
	R	70	81	15.7
Lysholm	L	60	93	55
	R	65	79	21.5
Tegner	L	2	6	200
	R	5	5	0

Case 2

The patient is a 59-year-old woman with a progressive history of more than 10 years of bilateral knee pain. The patient had no previous bracing, surgery, therapy, or dislocations. She complained of bilateral grinding within the front of both knees. She described severe limitations in her ability to perform activities of daily living and recreational activities. She has a sedentary job.

Preoperative physical examination showed symmetric findings bilaterally. Range of motion was 0° to 135°. She had painful arc of motion with palpable and audible crepitance from 30° thru 135°. Pain limited the patient from doing a one-leg step up without an assistive device. Marked pain was noted with patellofemoral compression. The Q angle was 10°, and the patient had symmetric quad atrophy compared with other lower extremity muscle groups. The knee was stable, and she had no increase in pain with patellar lateral apprehension testing. The medial and lateral compartments were unremarkable, and the knee was stable without effusion. Preoperative radiographs showed advanced isolated patellofemoral arthrosis with lateral patellar subluxation.

Index procedure

The patient underwent right knee arthroscopy with intra-articular debridement, arthroscopic lateral release, open patellofemoral HemiCAP resurfacing, and medial retinacular plication. There was minimal blood loss, and the surgery was conducted on an outpatient basis. The patient was noted to have 110° of flexion the first postoperative week, with 135° degrees after the third postoperative week. At last follow-up, 3 months after the procedure, the patient reported "great

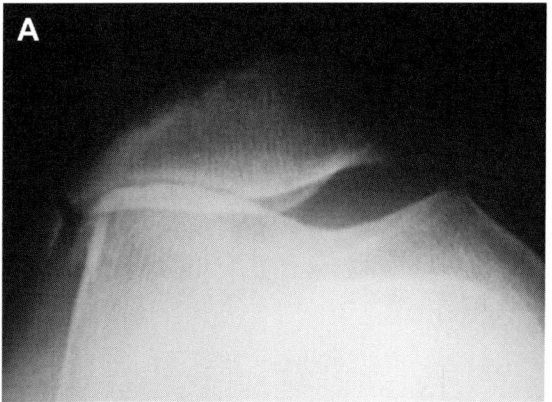 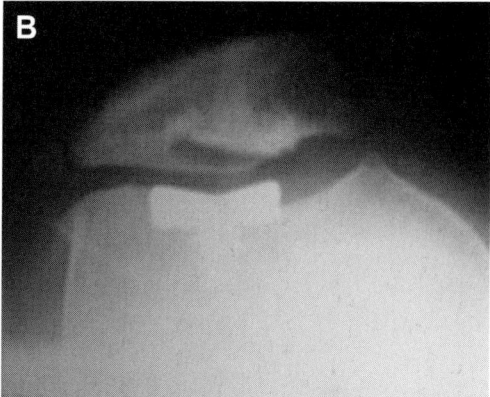

Fig. 8. (*A*) Case 1, Merchant preoperative x-ray. (*B*) Case 1, Merchant postoperative x-ray after patellar and trochlear HemiCAP resurfacing with lateral release and medial retinacular plication. (Note: improved patellofemoral tracking alignment).

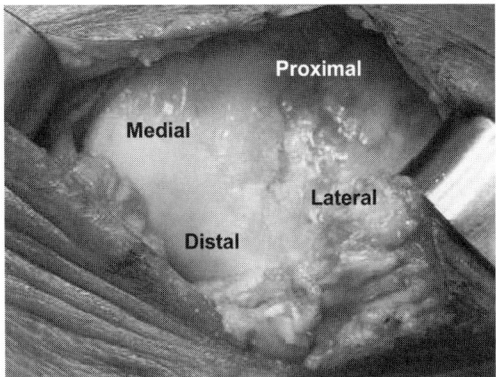

Fig. 9. Case 1; mini open view, trochlear pathology.

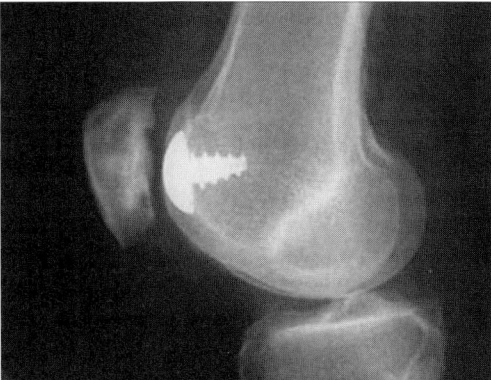

Fig. 11. Case 1; postoperative lateral radiograph after patellar and trochlear HemiCAP resurfacing.

pain relief and near-normal range of motion" (Table 2).

Currently the patient is pending contralateral surgery as she waits to accumulate time off from work to accommodate the procedure and postoperative recovery (Fig. 12).

Discussion

Many investigators have stressed the importance of prosthetic design factors to improve outcomes of isolated patellofemoral arthroplasty [3,14,15,29–31]. A wider selection available on the market today and improved prosthetic geometry have led to increased interest in unicompartmental arthroplasty of the patellofemoral joint. In conventional onlay patellofemoral arthroplasty, the implant geometry typically dictates the new joint surface, imparting nonnative geometry. Therefore, HemiCAP inlay resurfacing may have significant intrinsic advantages in patients with patellofemoral defects surrounded by relatively healthy articular cartilage margins and proper, or improved, extensor mechanism alignment.

Three-dimensional intraoperative mapping of the joint curvatures, preparation of a shallow implant bed, and placement of matching contoured articular inlay components provide preservation of healthy articular cartilage and valuable bone stock, avoid the risk of overstuffing the joint, and may keep the biomechanics of the patellofemoral joint unaltered. Soft tissues and extensor mechanism maintain their original tension, which may aid in postoperative recovery and strengthening. Prosthetic stability and fixation are embedded into the overall joint surface, providing a theoretic advantage for implant stability in comparison with exposed onlay prosthetic devices.

Bone cuts, as typically performed during conventional patellofemoral arthroplasty, are avoided using the described technique. This is

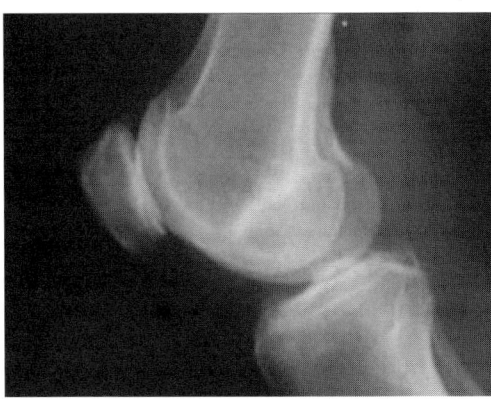

Fig. 10. Case 1; preoperative lateral radiograph.

Table 2
Case 2: outcomes measures for right knee with 3 months of follow-up

Outcomes score	Preoperative assessment	Last follow-up assessment	Percent improvement
SF-36 (Physical)	25.9	41.8	61.4
IKDC	30.9	66.7	115.8
Fulkerson knee score	31	86	177.4
Lysholm	29	88	203.4
Tegner	1	2	100

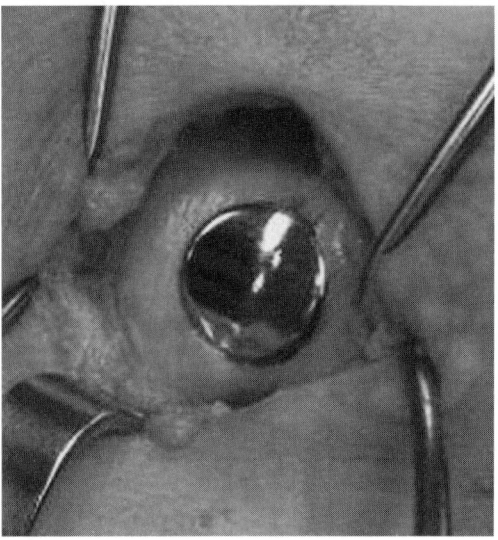

Fig. 12. Case 2; trochlear resurfacing component in place.

not only important in the context of minimal impact on joint biomechanics but also in the background of future revision surgery, should the need arise.

In particular, younger and active patients with isolated patellofemoral degeneration may benefit the most from a cartilage and bone stock–preserving procedure. At the same time, older patients with more compromised or fragile health may derive a medical advantage from focal resurfacing through minimized surgical dissection, shorter procedure time, and a reduction in potential blood loss.

Primary implant stability is provided through the fixation stud anchored into the distal trochlea, connected with an articular component via taper interlock, which is seated in a precision-reamed shallow implant bed. Because of the similarities in implant design and material with undersurface titanium coverage and titanium fixation component, a comparison to the goat study of Kirker-Head and colleagues [23] for focal femoral resurfacing may be suitable. The investigators have shown secondary stability with new trabecular bone abutted to the underside of the articular component and around the fixation stud without any evidence of a residual adverse inflammatory reaction to the implant or any indication of subchondral cyst formation in the medullary tissue surrounding the prosthesis.

High loads and complex patellofemoral joint surface geometry are challenging for biologic resurfacing methods. Therefore, patients who have not responded to such treatment options, or are not amenable because of advanced age or postimplantation requirements with prolonged protected physical therapy, may benefit from a stable prosthetic inlay construct with immediate primary fixation that allows for accelerated rehabilitation.

Patellofemoral malalignment reduces the contact area between patella and trochlea, thus, reducing the load-bearing surface over which forces from the extensor mechanism are transmitted to the femur [32].

Although overall patellofemoral joint reactive forces remain the same, the reduced contact area leads to focally elevated joint stresses [33–37]. Correction of malalignment in combination with a load-sharing congruent inlay resurfacing may help in normalizing patellofemoral joint kinematics and will have advantages for implant survivorship.

Becher and colleagues [27] found no significant differences in peak contact pressure for flush HemiCAP implantation in the femoral condyle when compared with the normal, untreated joint. Future basic science investigations will need to establish scientific evidence for patellofemoral joint kinematics after HemiCAP resurfacing.

The HemiCAP patellofemoral resurfacing procedure is highly reproducible and therefore has a short learning curve. Nevertheless, poor patient selection, technical errors, residual soft tissue imbalance, and continuation of patellofemoral or tibiofemoral degeneration may have a negative impact on clinical outcomes.

Intermediate and long-term clinical outcomes are required to show the benefits of this technology and allow for comparison with other patellofemoral treatment options including conventional arthroplasty. Future increase in prosthetic surface coverage will make the HemiCAP patellofemoral resurfacing technology accessible to a wider range of patients with more diffuse and degenerative cartilage defects of the patellofemoral joint.

Summary

Distal patellofemoral inlay resurfacing with the HemiCAP technology is a novel treatment option. It is indicated for patients with relatively localized defects or degeneration limited to the distal femoral trochlear and patellar. The native joint surface geometry is intraoperatively mapped for inset surface components with matching offsets. The trochlear and patellar prostheses are implanted congruent to the surrounding articular surface, conveying intrinsic stability. Proper patellofemoral tracking must be present or should be addressed in concurrent procedures. This patellofemoral resurfacing system may provide advantages for joint preservation, biomechanics, and component fixation when compared with traditional onlay arthroplasty. This initial report outlines theoretic concepts and surgical technique and provides case reports.

References

[1] McAlindon TE, Snow S, Cooper C, et al. Radiographic pattern of osteo-arthritis of the knee joint in the community: the importance of the patellofemoral joint. Ann Rheum Dis 1992;51:844-9.

[2] Davis AP, Vince AS, Shepstone L, et al. The Radiologic prevalence of patellofemoral osteoarthritis. Clin Orthop 2002;402:206-12.

[3] Blazina ME, Fox JM, Del Pizzo W, et al. Patellofemoral replacement. Clin Orthop Relat Res 1979;144: 98-102.

[4] Arciero RA, Toomey HE. Patellofemoral arthroplasty: a three- to nine-year follow-up study. Clin Orthop Relat Res 1988;236:60-71.

[5] Cartier P, Sanouiller JL, Grelsamer R. Patellofemoral arthroplasty: 2-12- year follow-up study. J Arthroplasty 1990;5:49-55.

[6] De Winter WE, Feith R, van Loon CJ. The Richards type II patellofemoral arthroplasty: 26 cases followed for 1-20 years. Acta Orthop Scand 2001;72: 487-90.

[7] Krajca-Radcliffe JB, Coker TP. Patellofemoral arthroplasty: A 2- to 18-year follow up study. Clin Orthop Relat Res 1996;330:143-51.

[8] Argenson JN, Flecher X, Parratte S, et al. Patellofemoral arthroplasty: an update. Clin Orthop Relat Res 2005;440:50-3.

[9] Lonner JH. Patellofemoral arthroplasty. J Am Acad Orthop Surg 2007;15(8):495-506.

[10] Curl WW, Krome J, Gordon ES, et al. Cartilage injuries: a review of 31,516 knee arthroscopies. Arthroscopy 1997;13(4):456-60.

[11] Fulkerson JP. Alternatives to patellofemoral arthroplasty. Clin Orthop Relat Res 2005;436:76-80.

[12] Gomoll AH, Minas T, Farr J, et al. Treatment of chondral defects in the patellofemoral joint. J Knee Surg 2006;19(4):285-95.

[13] Mandelbaum B, Browne JE, Fu F, et al. Treatment outcomes of autologous chondrocyte implantation for full-thickness articular cartilage defects of the trochlea. Am J Sports Med 2007;35(6):915-21.

[14] Leadbetter WB, Ragland PS, Mont MA. The appropriate use of patellofemoral arthroplasty: an analysis of reported indications, contraindications, and failures. Clin Orthop Relat Res 2005;436:91-9.

[15] Leadbetter WB, Seyler TM, Ragland PS, et al. Indications, contraindications, and pitfalls of patellofemoral arthroplasty. J Bone Joint Surg Am 2006; 88(Suppl 4):122-37.

[16] Mont MA, Haas S, Mullick T, et al. Total knee arthroplasty for patellofemoral arthritis. J Bone Joint Surg Am 2002;84(11):1977-81.

[17] Parvizi J, Stuart MJ, Pagnano MW, et al. Total knee arthroplasty in patients with isolated patellofemoral arthritis. Clin Orthop Relat Res 2001;392:147-52.

[18] Grelsamer RP, Stein DA. Patellofemoral arthritis. J Bone Joint Surg Am 2006;88(8):1849-60.

[19] Federico DJ, Reider B. Results of isolated patellar debridement for patellofemoral pain in patients with normal patellar alignment. Am J Sports Med 1997;25:663-9.

[20] Hangody L, Fules P. Autologous osteochondral mosaicplasty for the treatment of full-thickness defects of weight-bearing joints: ten years of experimental and clinical research. J Bone Joint Surg Am 2003;85(Suppl 2):25-32.

[21] Minas T, Bryant T. The role of autologous chondrocyte implantation in the patellofemoral joint. Clin Orthop Relat Res 2005;436:30-9.

[22] Nakagawa K, Wada Y, Minamide M, et al. Deterioration of longterm clinical results after the Elmslie-Trillat procedure for islocation of the patella. J Bone Joint Surg [Br] 2002;84:861-4.

[23] Kirker-Head CA, Van Sickle DC, Ek SW, et al. Safety of, and biological and functional response to, a novel metallic implant for the management of focal full-thickness cartilage defects: preliminary assessment in an animal model out to 1 year. J Orthop Res 2006;24(5):1095-108.

[24] Burks JB. Implant arthroplasty of the first metatarsalphalangeal joint. Clin Podiatr Med Surg 2006; 23(4):725-31.

[25] Jäger M, Begg MJ, Krauspe R. Partial hemi-resurfacing of the hip joint–a new approach to treat local osteochondral defects? [review]. Biomed Tech (Berl) 2006;51(5-6):371-6.

[26] Scalise JJ, Miniaci A, Iannotti JP. Resurfacing arthroplasty of the humerus: indications, surgical technique, and clinical results. Techniques in Shoulder and Elbow Surgery 2007;8(3):152-60.

[27] Becher C, Huber R, Thermann H, et al. Effects of a contoured articular prosthetic device on tibiofemoral peak contact pressure: a biomechanical study. Knee Surg Sports Traumatol Arthrosc 2008;16(1):56-63.

[28] Baldini A, Anderson JA, Cerulli-Mariani P, et al. Patellofemoral evaluation after total knee arthroplasty. Validation of a new weight-bearing axial radiographic view. J Bone Joint Surg Am 2007;89(8): 1810-7.

[29] Lonner JH. Patellofemoral arthroplasty. Pros, cons, and design considerations. Clin Orthop Relat Res 2004;428:158-65.

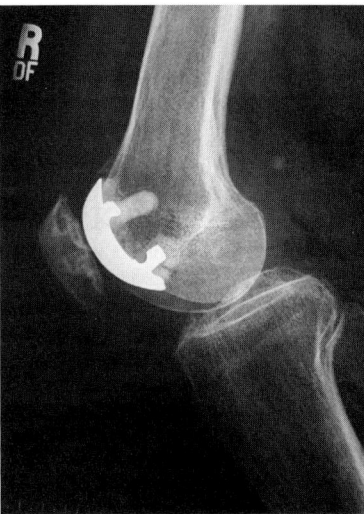

Fig. 1. Lateral radiograph of an inlay trochlear component (Lubinus prosthesis). The obtuse design required flexion of the component, leaving it prominent proximally. (*Reproduced from* Lonner JH. Patellofemoral arthroplasty: pros, cons, and design considerations. Clin Orthop Relat Res 2004;428:158–65; with permission.)

The proximal extension of the trochlear flange on the anterior femur also differs between products (Figs. 6 and 7). Onlay implants are typically designed to extend considerably more proximal than the articular margin of the trochlear so that the patellar component articulates entirely with the trochlear component in extension (see Fig. 2B). On the other hand, inlay designs, like the Lubinus and LCS components, and custom designs, like the Kinamed, do not extend proximal to the articular cartilage margin of the trochlea. The patellar prosthesis in those latter designs therefore articulates with the natural anterior femoral surface in full extension before it transitions onto the trochlear prosthesis. This predisposes these designs to catching and snapping in the initial 30 degrees of flexion, particularly if the trochlear prosthesis is flexed or offset anteriorly [4]. The problem is compounded by components with greater trochlear constraint in the axial plane such as the Lubinus, LCS, and Richards Mod I and II designs. Other implants have found a balance between constraint and freedom within the trochlear groove that is more forgiving in extension than other systems (Fig. 2A; see Fig. 2C).

Implants differ in the thickness of the components as well. The traditional inlay-type devices are thinner than the onlay devices, since the philosophy of those designs is to minimize removal of bone. Some onlay and custom implants have a thicker component in an attempt to restore trochlear offset [9,12]. Occasionally this may stuff the patellofemoral joint and predispose to patellofemoral pain from soft tissue irritation or increased loads. Despite the attraction to the conservative bone resection with inlay designs, their clinical performance tends to be less predictable than onlay devices [1–10] and revision can be performed with each style of patellofemoral implant [13,14].

Some components are asymmetric, to theoretically optimize patella tracking; others are symmetric. For instance, the Avon component (Stryker, Mahwah, NJ) is symmetric, with one trochlear geometry for both right and left knees. An analysis of radiographs shows that the coronal (varus-valgus) orientation of the component varies from patient to patient, although the clinical implications of this are unclear (Figs. 8–10). The varus-valgus orientation of the component is determined by the fit of the intercondylar tail of the trochlear component relative to the articular surfaces of the medial and lateral femoral condyles, since it must be flush. This variability in coronal orientation may impact patella tracking, particularly in cases where there is considerable vector toward the lateral side of the knee. There have been cases of squeaking observed with both the Avon component and the Lubinus, which may be related to eccentric tracking of the patella on the trochlea and asymmetric loads on the component that have not been observed with a more asymmetric design and enhanced trochlear tracking angle, in the author's experience (see Fig. 2A).

As stated earlier, some trochlear designs are an inlay-type, others are an onlay-type component. The former design is inset into the trochlea and tends to be more bone conserving; the latter is implanted flush with the anterior surface of the femoral cortex and removes the entire anterior trochlear surface. However, given the variability in distal anterior femoral morphology, inlayed components often do not accurately mate with the articular geometry of the trochlear region of the femur, resulting in offset on any of its edges. This typically results in patella catching on the trochlear component, either proximally as the knee proceeds from extension to flexion, or distally as the knee proceeds from deep flexion to extension. The onlay device is more suitable for a larger variation in trochlear geometries. Unlike the inlay designs, it can be applied in patients with

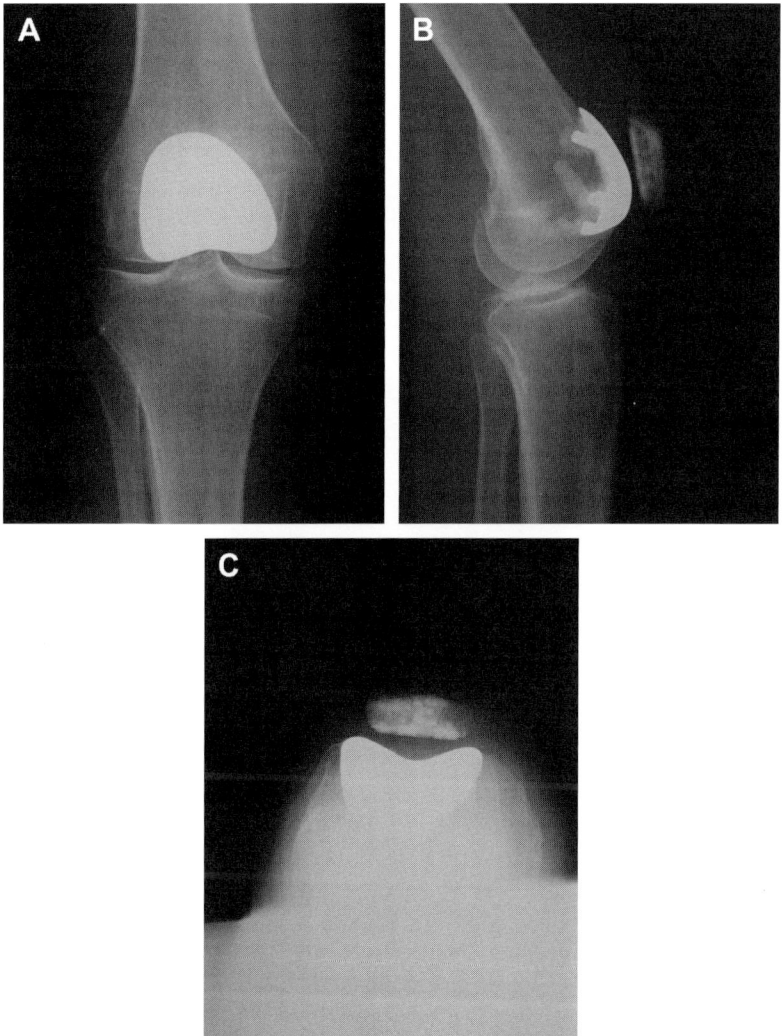

Fig. 2. Anteroposterior (AP), lateral, and axial radiographs of the Zimmer Gender Solutions PFJ. These radiographs demonstrate the valgus tracking angle of the component (*A*), optimized sagittal radius of curvature (*B*), and broad coverage provided anteriorly (*C*).

trochlear dysplasia without risk of having the component sit proud relative to the surrounding articular cartilage. It is this author's opinion that trying to inset a trochlear component into the bone is analogous to implanting a potato chip onto the anterior aspect of the knee. If the two surfaces are geometrically mated then the outcome will be absolutely perfect. But if there is a mismatch, then there is an increased risk for relative component malalignment and malposition relative to the articular surfaces, which is why patella maltracking is more common with that style of implant.

Clinical results and complications by design

The first generation of implants, the Lubinus (Link, Hamburg, Germany) and the Richards Mod I and II (Smith Nephew Richards, Memphis, TN) had good and excellent results that ranged from 45% to 88% at short and midterm follow-up, with a high incidence of secondary surgeries necessary for correction of patellar instability and mechanical problems, such as the patella catching on the edges of the trochlear component [1–8]. Again, the relatively high tendency for patellofemoral complications with these implants were

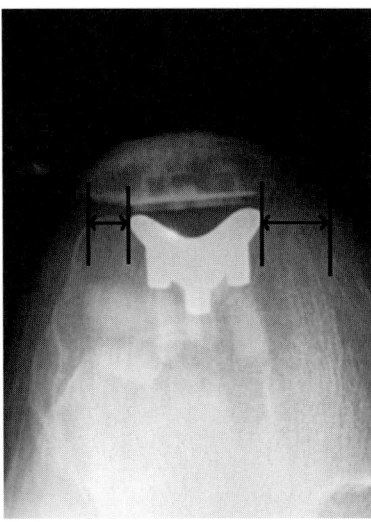

Fig. 3. Axial radiograph of a large-size Lubinus implant demonstrating how narrow the component is. The arrows demonstrate the extent of cartilage that is not covered by the prosthesis. (*Reproduced from* Lonner JH. Patellofemoral arthroplasty: pros, cons, and design considerations. Clin Orthop Relat Res 2004;428: 158–65; with permission.)

often erroneously attributed to poor patient selection, malposition, and soft tissue imbalance. However, these problems were likely most related to trochlear design features that put the patella at risk for maltracking [4]. The deep, constraining trochlear groove of the Richards Mod I and II implants predisposed to subtle maltracking and catching of the implant on the trochlear edges, requiring secondary surgeries in as many as 18% to

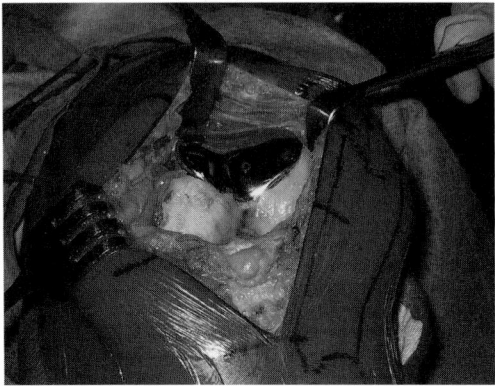

Fig. 4. Intraoperative photograph of the Zimmer Gender Solutions PFJ, demonstrating maximized coverage of the prepared bone anteriorly and a flush zone of transition where the edges contact the femoral condyles.

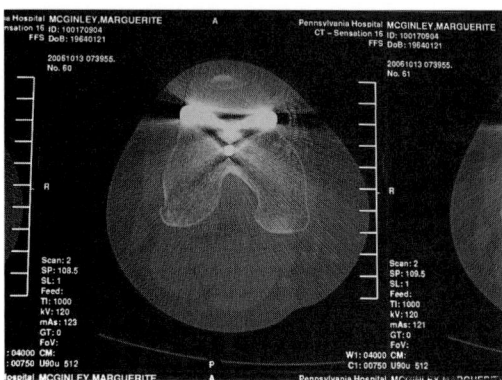

Fig. 5. Axial computed tomography scan of an extra-small-size Avon trochlear component on an averaged sized female who had some soft tissue crepitus after patellofemoral arthroplasty, demonstrating 1 to 2 mm of medial and lateral overhang.

27% of cases [15,16]. The Lubinus patellofemoral implant has also been associated with a high rate of reoperation for patellofemoral dysfunction. For instance, Tauro and colleagues [5] reported a need for revision to another patellofemoral arthroplasty (PFA) or total knee arthroplasty (TKA) in 28% of knees with that prosthesis, primarily for patellar maltracking. The authors reported trochlear malalignment or patellar

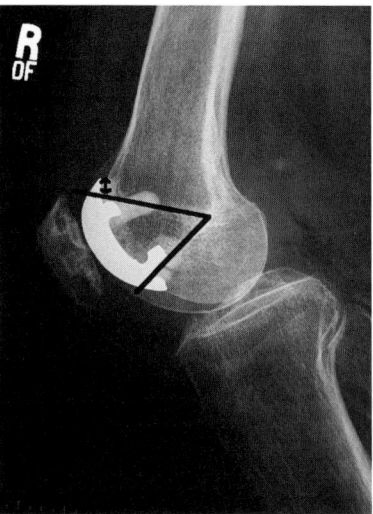

Fig. 6. Limited proximal extension of the Lubinus trochlear implant above the physeal scar predisposes to patellar tracking problems. (*Reproduced from* Lonner JH. Patellofemoral arthroplasty: pros, cons, and design considerations. Clin Orthop Relat Res 2004;428: 158–65; with permission.)

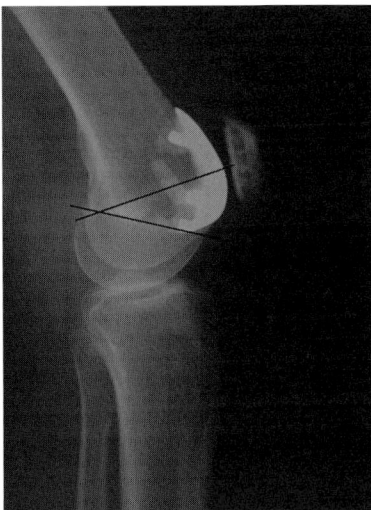

Fig. 7. Enhanced proximal extension of the anterior trochlear flange of the Zimmer Gender Solutions PFJ, well proximal to the physeal scar.

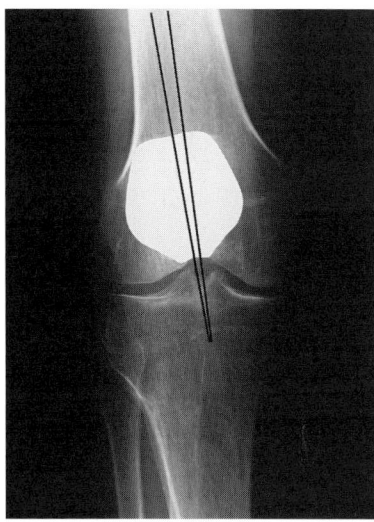

Fig. 9. AP radiograph after patellofemoral arthroplasty using the symmetric Avon design. The component is oriented in a relatively varus position relative to the anatomic axis of the femoral shaft.

maltracking in 32% of cases, although these were not always symptomatic. Another series reported the incidence of patellofemoral dysfunction, subluxation, catching, and substantial pain to be 17% with the Lubinus prosthesis [4].

Second-generation implants, namely the Autocentric (DePuy, Warsaw, IN), Avon (Stryker, Mahwah, NJ), and the LCS mobile bearing (DePuy), have had greater short- and midterm success, in the range of 84% to 96% good and excellent results [4,9,10,17], because of improved trochlear design features that substantially reduced the incidence of patella maltracking. For instance, the incidence of patellar maltracking is

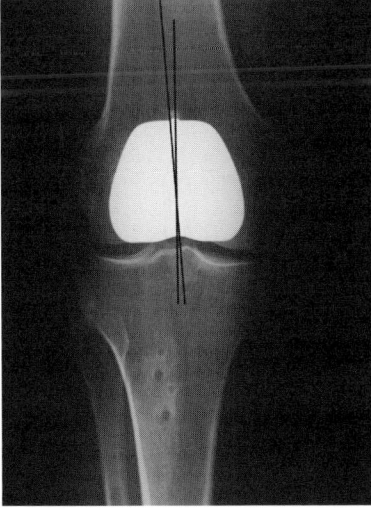

Fig. 8. AP radiograph after patellofemoral arthroplasty using the symmetric Avon design. The component is oriented in a neutral position relative to the mechanical axis of the femur.

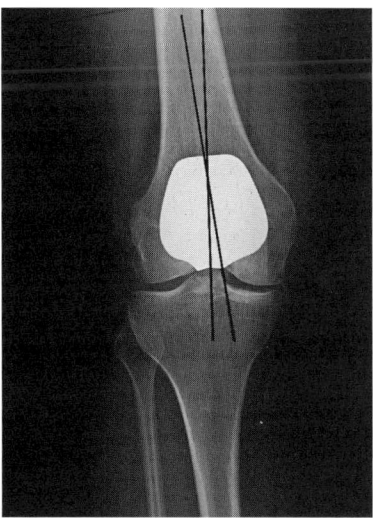

Fig. 10. AP radiograph after patellofemoral arthroplasty using the symmetric Avon design. The component is oriented in a relatively valgus position relative to the anatomic axis of the femoral shaft.

less than 1% with the second-generation design of the Avon trochlear implant [4,9]. The broad flange of the Avon has had some cases of trochlear overhang, resulting in soft tissue irritation and crepitus but only moderate and intermittent discomfort (see Fig. 5). Custom and contemporary implants have still greater prospects for improved patellofemoral performance, once again related primarily to improved trochlear design features, but also to availability of more sophisticated instrumentation that improves the accuracy of implantation (Figs. 11 and 12).

The Australian Orthopaedic Association, National Joint Replacement Registry, has provided insight into the experience with and outcomes after patellofemoral arthroplasty performed between 1999 and 2005. In that registry, 76.7% of the 675 patellofemoral arthroplasties performed in Australia were in women, usually in patients younger than 55 (38.4%) or between the ages of 55 and 64 (28.4%). The tendency for revision after patellofemoral arthroplasty varied between component types. For instance, in that series, the incidence of revision was 12.3% with the Richards Mod III, 7.3% with the Lubinus, 5.6% with the LCS, and 3.4% with the Avon, all systems typically available in the United States [18]. The registry does not clearly elucidate the mechanisms of failure and reasons for revision with each individual implant but the data does corroborate other studies that show a higher incidence of patellofemoral-related problems with some implants compared with others.

A study by Hendrix and colleagues [14] found that significant improvement can be obtained when revising one failed patellofemoral

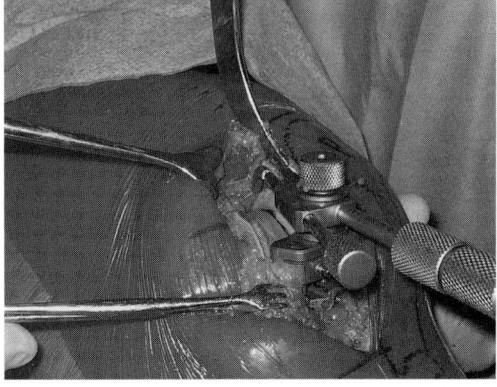

Fig. 11. Intraoperative photograph of a contemporary low-profile instrument for preparation of the anterior surface of the trochlea with an onlay technique.

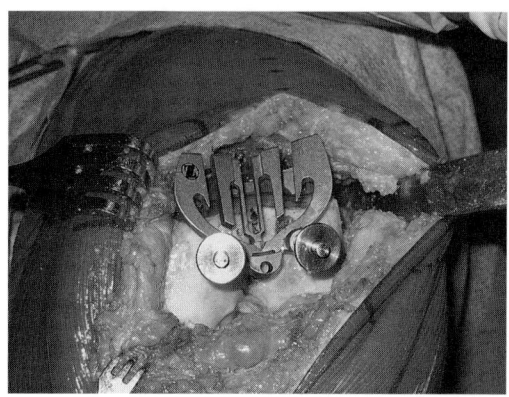

Fig. 12. Photograph of a contemporary low-profile milling device for preparation of the intercondylar surface of the distal femur.

arthroplasty design, which has been plagued by maltracking problems, to an alternate design with improved features for patellar tracking. In that series, 14 Lubinus implants in 14 knees were revised to the Avon system for component malposition, patella subluxation, polyethylene wear, or overstuffing. Mean Bristol knee scores improved from 58 (range 36 to 86) to 79 (range 38 to 100) ($P < .001$). The presence of mild tibiofemoral arthritis was predictive of a poorer outcome. At most recent follow-up, at a mean of 5 years following revision surgery, there were no cases of patellar subluxation wear or loosening.

Unique design features of the zimmer gender solutions PFJ

Recent experience with a more contemporary implant (Gender Solutions PFJ, Zimmer, Warsaw, IN) has demonstrated further improvement in outcomes and optimization of patella tracking. The Zimmer Gender Solutions PFJ is an asymmetric design that takes into consideration that the vast majority of PFA recipients are women. In all but its largest size, its trochlear groove angle is increased to accommodate the relatively high Q angle typical in women, as well as the common tendency for preoperative patellar subluxation in female patients who have patellofemoral arthritis. This design feature has enhanced patellar tracking and minimized the need for lateral release during the procedure. Additionally, because of the trochlear angle of this implant, radiographs have consistently shown valgus orientation of the femoral component and reduced the tendency for variability in the trochlear position in the coronal plane that has been observed with other implants (see Fig. 2A). The largest trochlear component, anticipated to be used primarily for larger male patients, has a slightly lower valgus tracking angle than the other sizes, to accommodate a typically lower Q angle in male patients. Incidentally, the largest trochlear implant is relatively thicker than the other sizes, to provide additional anterior trochlear offset and mechanical advantage in larger male patients. Perhaps as a result of the optimized trochlear tracking angle or the reduced thickness of the trochlear flange relative to other designs, there have been no reported cases of patellofemoral squeaking with this design that have been observed with other implants. The proximal extension of the trochlear component is increased such that the patella should be in contact with the trochlear prosthesis throughout the entire range of extension, except perhaps in some very unusual cases of extreme patella alta (see Fig. 7). The transitional point between the anterior trochlear flange and the intercondylar portion of the component has been refined so that the engagement of the patella is enhanced as the knee proceeds into flexion, increasing the arc of flexion before the lateral and medial edges of the patella component begin to articulate on the articular cartilage of the weight-bearing surfaces of the femoral condyles. The design of this implant also accommodates a unicompartmental arthroplasty, whether performed concurrently or staged, without encroachment of the two prosthetic surfaces. The implant has five sizes, which vary in all dimensions, but primarily in the mediolateral breadth of the implant. The expanse of size options has limited the risk of mediolateral component overhang and subsequent soft tissue crepitus that has been observed with other designs (found particularly in patients with smaller bones, representing the majority of recipients). The implant is an onlay design that requires a flush anterior cut tangential with the anterior femoral cortex. This was a necessary design feature to allow its routine use in patients who have dysplasia of the medial or lateral trochlear surfaces, so that the implant can be mated with all morphologies of the distal femur, which is not possible with inlay-type components. The sagittal radius of curvature mates accurately with the distal femoral radius of curvature that have been studied and encountered clinically. Additionally, the intercondylar tail of the component has been shortened compared with other designs and tucks into the bone to avoid impingement of the proximal pole of the patellar component as it moves onto the trochlear implant while the knee extends. The patellar component is a typical all-polyethylene modified dome that is perfectly suited to PFA, but that can also be retained if it is revised to a TKA.

In addition to the design features of this component, which have substantially improved patella tracking, instrumentation has been developed that is low profile, accurate, and conducive to less invasive surgical techniques. It offers the first fully instrumented system for patellofemoral arthroplasty. Early generation implants required freehand preparation of all of the bony surfaces, which contributed to inaccurate trochlear component alignment. Second-generation implants typically neither offered a means for preparing the distal femur for the intercondylar tail of the implant, nor were they amenable to more contemporary, less invasive surgical techniques, since they tended to be quite bulky. Furthermore, the Zimmer Gender Solutions PFJ incorporates a sophisticated milling system that ensures accurate preparation to the intercondylar region to accommodate the implant (see Fig. 12). This system has dramatically simplified the procedure and ensures anatomic mating of the implant to the articular surfaces of the transition zone. This milling system provides an effective means for addressing condylar variability and provides unique depth control and accuracy of preparation of the transitional surfaces in this region, unlike the freehand techniques of other available systems.

Summary

Given recent improvements in patellofemoral arthroplasty design, early failures from patellofemoral maltracking will no longer occur to the extent that they had in the past. The implant design has been shown to impact clinical results and should play a role in component selection when opting to perform patellofemoral arthroplasty for a patient. More sophisticated instrumentation will also facilitate the surgical procedure and improve the accuracy of implantation, even through less invasive surgical approaches.

References

[1] Arciero R, Toomey H. Patellofemoral arthroplasty. A three to nine year follow-up study. Clin Orthop Relat Res 1988;236:60–71.
[2] Krajca-Radcliffe JB, Coker TP. Patellofemoral arthroplasty. A 2- to 18-year followup study. Clin Orthop Relat Res 1996;330:143–51.

[3] Board TN, Mahmood A, Ryan WG, et al. The Lubinus patellofemoral arthroplasty: a series of 17 cases. Arch Orthop Trauma Surg 2004;124(5):285–7.

[4] Lonner JH. Patellofemoral arthroplasty: pros, cons, and design considerations. Clin Orthop Relat Res 2004;428:158–65.

[5] Tauro B, Ackroyd CE, Newman JH, et al. The Lubinus patellofemoral arthroplasty. A 5 to 10 year prospective study. J Bone Joint Surg Br 2001;83(5):696–701.

[6] Smith AM, Peckett WR, Butler-Manuel PA, et al. Treatment of patello-femoral arthritis using the Lubinus patello-femoral arthroplasty: a retrospective review. Knee 2002;9(1):27–30.

[7] Blazina ME, Fox JM, Del Pizzo W, et al. Patellofemoral replacement. Clin Orthop Relat Res 1979;144(7):98–106.

[8] Cartier P, Sanouiller JL, Khefacha A. Long-term results with the first patellofemoral prosthesis. Clin Orthop Relat Res 2005;436(7):47–54.

[9] Ackroyd CE, Newman JH, Evans R, et al. The Avon patellofemoral arthroplasty. Five-year survivorship and functional results. J Bone Joint Surg Br 2007;89B:310–5.

[10] Argenson JNA, Flecher X, Parratte S, et al. Patellofemoral arthroplasty: an update. Clin Orthop Relat Res 2005;440(11):50–3.

[11] Lonner JH. Patellofemoral arthroplasty. J Am Acad Orthop Surg 2007;15:495–506.

[12] Sisto DJ, Sarin VK. Custom patellofemoral arthroplasty of the knee. J Bone Joint Surg Am 2006;88A:1475–80.

[13] Lonner JH, Jasko JG, Booth RE Jr. Revision of a failed patellofemoral arthroplasty to a total knee replacement. J Bone Joint Surg Am 2006;88(11):2337.

[14] Hendrix MRG, Ackroyd CE, Lonner JH. Revision patellofemoral arthroplasty: three to seven year follow up period. J Arthrop 2007, in press.

[15] de Winter WE, Feith R, van Loon CJ. The Richards type II patellofemoral arthroplasty: 26 cases followed for 1–20 years. Acta Orthop Scand 2001;72:487–90.

[16] Kooijman HJ, Driesen AP, van Horn JR. Long-term results of patellofemoral arthroplasty. A report of 56 arthroplasties with 17 years of follow-up. J Bone Joint Surg Br 2003;85(6):836–40.

[17] Merchant AC. Early results with a total patellofemoral joint replacement arthroplasty prosthesis. J Arthrop 2004;19:829–36.

[18] Australian Orthopaedic Association National Joint Replacement Registry. Available at: http://www.aoa.org.au/docs/njrrrep06.pdf. Accessed April 30, 2008.

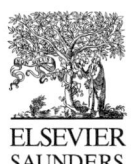

Patellofemoral Arthroplasty with a Customized Trochlear Prosthesis

Domenick J. Sisto, MD[a],*, Vineet K. Sarin, PhD[b]

[a]Los Angeles Orthopaedic Institute, 4955 Van Nuys Boulevard, Suite 615, Sherman Oaks, CA 91403, USA
[b]Kinamed Incorporated, 820 Flynn Road, Camarillo, CA 93012, USA

It has been estimated that isolated patellofemoral disease affects up to 11% of men and 24% of women who have painful arthritis of the knee joint [1]. Although conservative therapies and non-arthroplasty surgical treatments for isolated patellofemoral disease are well known [2], their effectiveness in treating the severely degenerated patellofemoral joint has been limited, especially in young, active patients. By contrast, it has been shown that total knee arthroplasty can provide excellent results for the treatment of isolated patellofemoral disease in elderly patients [3], but it is believed widely that total knee arthroplasty is not appropriate for patients under the age of 55 years. For these reasons, interest in patellofemoral arthroplasty has grown substantially in recent years.

A number of investigators have reported on the results of patellofemoral arthroplasty, with varying degrees of success (Table 1). These inconsistent results have contributed to controversy about the effectiveness of patellofemoral arthroplasty. Based on the collective historical experience with patellofemoral arthroplasty, failures generally are thought to be caused by a combination of inappropriate patient selection, prosthesis design, and surgical technique [18]. This article reviews the design rationale, clinical experience, and surgical technique of a unique approach to patellofemoral arthroplasty that incorporates a customized trochlear prosthesis designed to fit the individual patient's patellofemoral groove.

Design rationale

The customized trochlear prosthesis does not require femoral bone resection because CT modeling is used to model an exact fit to the femoral trochlear anatomy of the individual patient. The customized trochlear prosthesis is designed to approximate normal patellofemoral kinematics by re-establishing the alignment and depth of the trochlear groove and to improve quadriceps function by repositioning the patella anteriorly. The distal margin of the trochlear prosthesis is designed to rest 3 to 5 mm proximal to the apex of the femoral intercondylar notch. The prosthesis has a thickened lateral border to compensate for bone loss along the lateral edge of the trochlear groove and to provide congruency and tracking stability with the patellar implant. The thickened implant border does not anteriorize the patella because the anterior position of a given patella is defined by the thickness of the femoral implant's trochlear groove. The customized femoral prosthesis appears thick on lateral radiographs because the radiograph is a two-dimensional projection of a complex three-dimensional "saddle-like" shape whose functional thickness is obscured by its lateral border.

The customized trochlear prosthesis is designed to restore the anterior position of the normal, non-degenerated patella. The thickness of normal articular cartilage is approximately 4 to 5 mm on the patella and 2 to 3 mm in the trochlea, yielding a combined total cartilage thickness of 6 to 8 mm [19]. The customized trochlear prosthesis typically is 2 to 5 mm thick along the tracking arc of the patella. The maximal thickness along the tracking arc of the patella is a function of native trochlear groove depth (ie, thinner implants are

* Corresponding author.
E-mail address: laortho1@yahoo.com (D.J. Sisto).

Table 1
Published results of patellofemoral arthroplasty

Study	N	Follow-up (years)	Implant (manufacturer)	Salient results
Ackroyd and Chir [4]	306	2–5	Avon (Stryker, Allendale, NJ)	87% not revised and complication-free
Arciero and Toomey [5]	25	3–9	Blazina II (Richards, Memphis, TN) and CFS (Wright, Arlington, TN)	72% good or excellent; 12% revised
Argenson et al [6]	66	2–10	Autocentric (Medinov, Roanne, France)	85% not revised
Argenson et al [7]	66	12–20	Autocentric (DePuy, Warsaw, IN)	56% not revised
Blazina et al [8]	57	1–3.5	Blazina I & II (Richards)	78% "much improved"
Cartier et al [9]	72	2–12	Blazina II & III (Richards)	85% good or excellent; 8% mechanical complications
de Winter et al [10]	26	1–20	Blazina II (Richards)	61% good or excellent; 19% re-operation rate
Kooijman et al [11]	45	15–21	Blazina II (Richards)	62% not revised
Krajca-Radcliffe & Coker [12]	16	2–18	Bechtol I & II (Richards)	88% good or excellent; 19% re-operation rate
Lubinus [13]	14	0.5–2	Lubinus (Link, Hamburg, Germany)	"All improved"
Merchant [14]	15	2.2–5.5	LCS (DePuy)	93% good or excellent on ADL scale
Sisto & Sarin [15]	25	2.7–9.9	Custom (Kinamed)	100% good or excellent; no revisions or complications
Smith et al [16]	45	0.5–7.5	Lubinus (Link)	64% good or excellent; 19% revised
Tauro et al [17]	62	5–10	Lubinus (Link)	45% "satisfactory"; 28% revised

associated with shallower grooves). The thinner implants are designed specifically to avoid overstuffing the more dysplastic trochleas. Coupled with an anatomic restoration of the patella, the extensor lever arm is intended to be unchanged from the normal, healthy condition. If concerns about overstuffing persist, accommodations can be made by resecting more bone on the patellar side or by selecting a thinner patellar implant.

The precise fit achieved by the customized approach to patellofemoral arthroplasty is illustrated best by examining the customized trochlear prostheses that are designed for individual femurs of varying shape (Fig. 1A–D). Despite considerable variations in the alignment, shape, and depth of these native trochlear grooves, all the customized trochlear prostheses are adapted precisely to the bony contours of the native femur and conform to the patellofemoral articulation without overhang into the intercondylar notch.

Indications and contraindications

The indications and contraindications for patellofemoral arthroplasty have been summarized in detail by Leadbetter and colleagues [20]. Indications include but are not limited to

- Degenerative or posttraumatic osteoarthritis limited to the patellofemoral joint, so that medial and lateral Ahlback [21] scores are less than or equal to 1 point
- Severe symptoms affecting daily activity referable to patellofemoral joint degeneration unresponsive to lengthy nonoperative treatment and conservative procedures
- Patellofemoral malalignment/dysplasia-induced degeneration with or without instability
- Contraindications include but are not limited to
- Medial and lateral tibiofemoral compartment Ahlback scores greater than 1 point
- The lack of an attempt at nonoperative care or to rule out other sources of pain
- Systemic inflammatory arthropathy
- Uncorrected patellofemoral instability or malalignment

No indications or contraindications are associated specifically with the customized approach to patellofemoral arthroplasty.

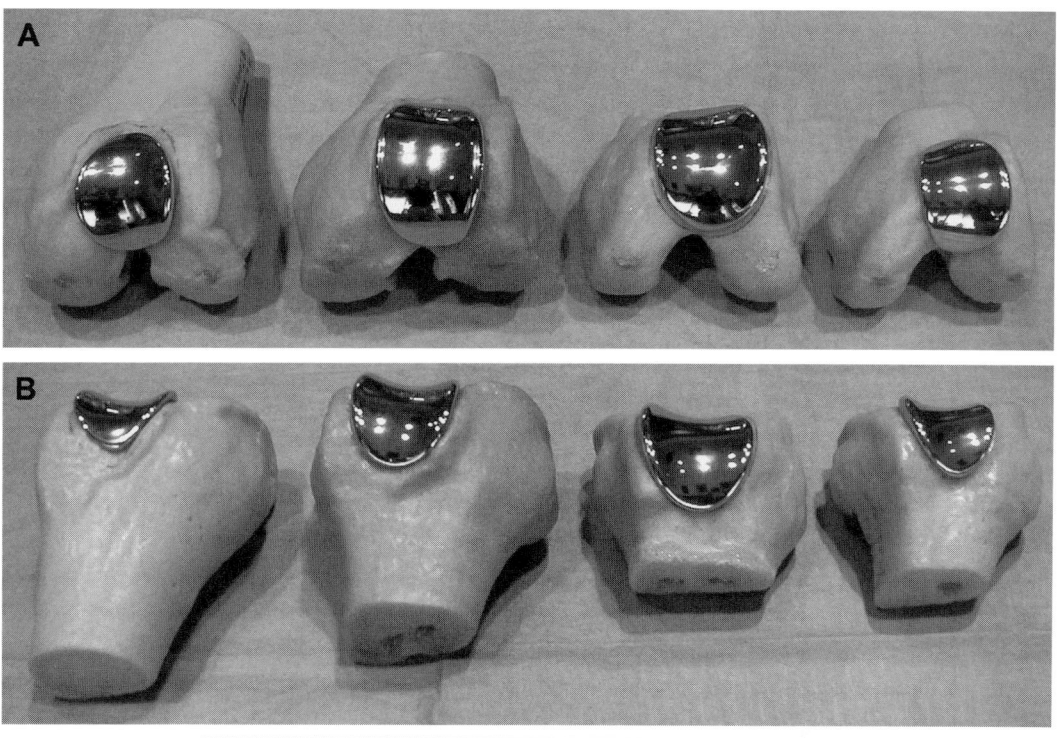
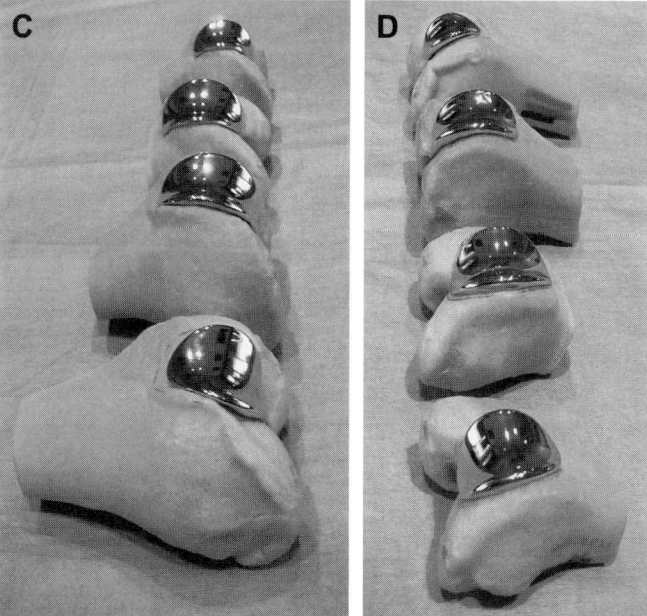

Fig. 1. (*A*) Variation in geometry of four trochlear grooves and precise fit of the customized trochlear prostheses in anterior view. (*B*) Precise fit of the customized prostheses at the top of the trochlear groove and build-up of lateral border thickness for increasing patella-tracking stability. Views of (*C*) lateral and (*D*) medial aspects show precise adaptation of the prostheses in the sagittal plane.

Clinical experience

The authors previously reported on the results of patellofemoral arthroplasty using a customized trochlear prosthesis and an off-the-shelf patella button prosthesis [15]. Twenty-five patellofemoral arthroplasties (3 bilateral) were performed in 22 patients for the treatment of isolated patellofemoral arthritis. There were 16 women (2 had bilateral arthroplasties) and 6 men (1 had bilateral arthroplasty) with a mean age of 45 years at surgery. Seventeen patients (19 knees) had had a prior surgical procedure on the knee. The mean preoperative Knee Society functional and objective scores were 49 points and 52 points, respectively. At a mean follow-up of 73 months postoperatively (range, 32–119 months), all 25 implants were in place (Fig. 2A–C) and were functioning well.

There were 18 excellent results and 7 good results according to the Knee Society scoring system. The mean Knee Society functional and objective scores were 89 points and 91 points, respectively. No patient had required additional surgery or had component loosening. The patients included in this study were monitored for an additional 30 months. All maintained their good to excellent Knee Society Score status without need for additional knee surgery.

Surgical technique

The surgical technique for patellofemoral arthroplasty using a customized trochlear prosthesis has been described previously in detail [22]. Because the customized trochlear prosthesis is

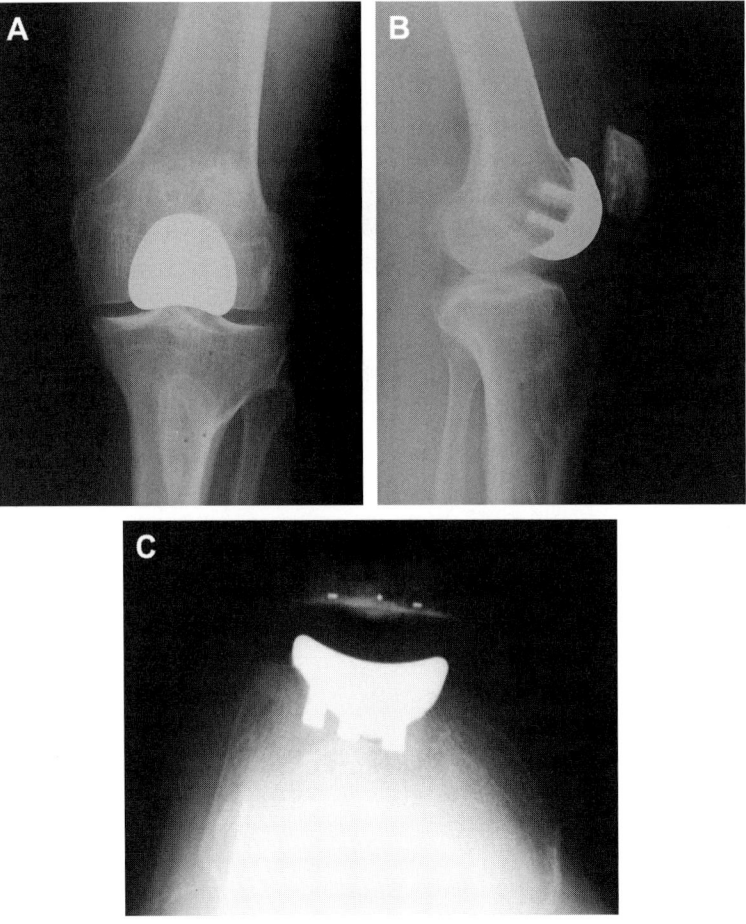

Fig. 2. Postoperative (*A*) anteroposterior, (*B*) lateral, and (*C*) Merchant-view radiographs reveal proper position of the customized patellofemoral prosthesis. (*From* Sisto DJ, Sarin VK. Custom patellofemoral arthroplasty of the knee: surgical technique. J Bone Joint Surg [Am] 2007;89(Suppl 2, Part 2):223; with permission.)

designed from CT data, the prosthesis fits precisely against the subchondral bone of the femoral trochlear groove, virtually eliminating the trade-off between alignment and fit that is common with off-the-shelf patellofemoral prostheses. Moreover, because the fit and alignment of the customized trochlear prosthesis is defined preoperatively, there is no need for intramedullary instrumentation or bone resection.

A CT scan of the patient's distal femur is performed according to the specific instructions provided by the manufacturer of the customized trochlear prosthesis (Kinamed, Camarillo, California). The surgeon receives a CT-reconstructed bone model for review before the surgery. Any planned osteophyte removal is communicated to the prosthesis manufacturer by physically performing the planned removal on the bone model and returning the model to the manufacturer before final prosthesis design.

After the femoral trochlea is exposed and the patella is everted (Fig. 3), a customized marking template and drill-guide is used to mark the perimeter for cartilage removal (Fig. 4). Because the CT scan models bone only, proper fit of the prosthesis is achieved by using a curette to excise any articular cartilage inside the marked perimeter (Fig. 5). The customized drill-guide then is used to drill three holes for the pegs of the prosthesis (Fig. 6). After the trochlear groove has been

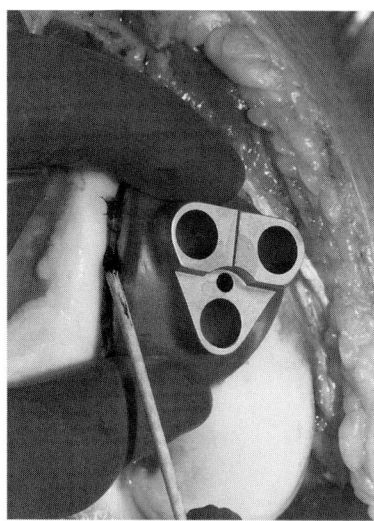

Fig. 4. The customized marking template and drill-guide is used to mark the perimeter for cartilage removal. (*Adapted from* Sisto DJ, Sarin VK. Custom patellofemoral arthroplasty of the knee: surgical technique. J Bone Joint Surg [Am] 2007;89(Suppl 2, Part 2):217; with permission.)

prepared (Fig. 7), the customized trochlear prosthesis is trial-fitted by placing the prosthesis pegs into the drilled holes and finding its natural fit on the femoral trochlea (Fig. 8).

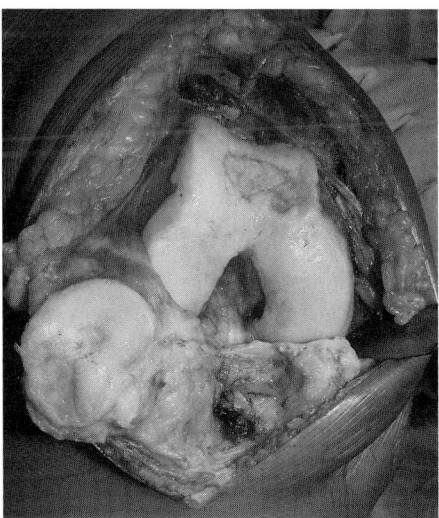

Fig. 3. Intraoperative view showing cartilage degeneration isolated to patellofemoral articulation. (*Adapted from* Sisto DJ, Sarin VK. Custom patellofemoral arthroplasty of the knee: surgical technique. J Bone Joint Surg [Am] 2007;89(Suppl 2, Part 2):216; with permission.)

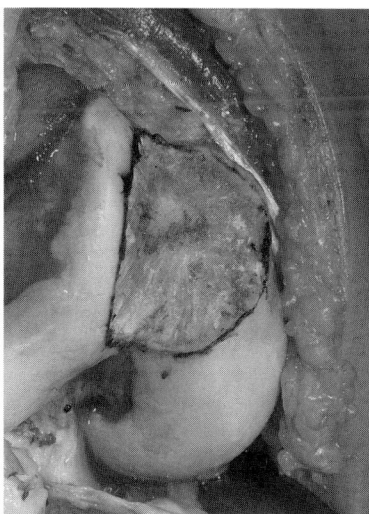

Fig. 5. Exposed subchondral bone inside the perimeter of the customized trochlear prosthesis. (*Adapted from* Sisto DJ, Sarin VK. Custom patellofemoral arthroplasty of the knee: surgical technique. J Bone Joint Surg [Am] 2007;89(Suppl 2, Part 2):219; with permission.)

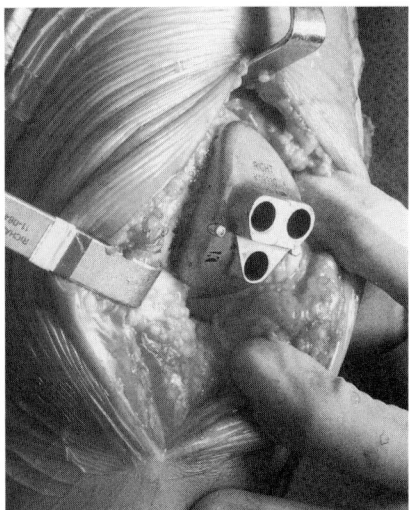

Fig. 6. Customized marking template and drill-guide affixed to the trochlear groove.

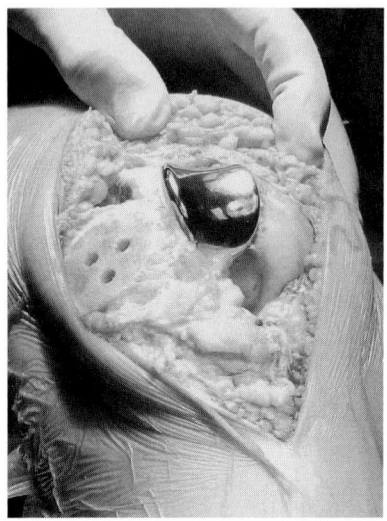

Fig. 8. Customized trochlear prosthesis trial-fitted in place. (*Image courtesy of* Robert Jackson MD, Provo, Utah.)

The customized trochlear prosthesis is designed to articulate with an off-the-shelf all-polyethylene domed patellar prosthesis. A dome-shaped patellar prosthesis (either inset or onlay) is selected so that the residual patella has a thickness of 15 mm or more after resection, thus maintaining the overall patellar thickness with the prosthesis in place. After a successful trial reduction, both the trochlear and patellar prostheses are cemented in place (Fig. 9). The patella is reduced to its anatomic position, and the knee is tested through a range of motion to be certain that patellar tracking is anatomic. Lateral retinacular releases are performed as indicated by the "no-thumb" test of patellar tracking.

Keys to success

The authors' experience with customized patellofemoral arthroplasty suggests several preoperative and intraoperative keys to success [22].

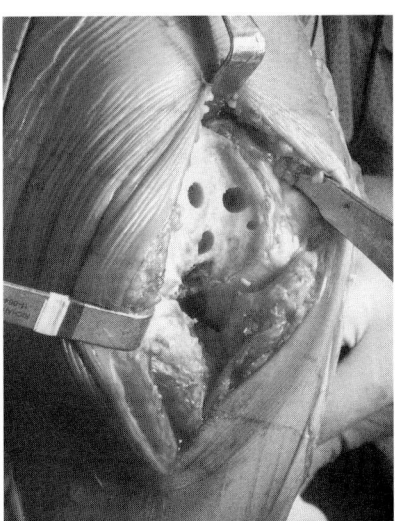

Fig. 7. Trochlear groove prepared to accept the customized trochlear prosthesis.

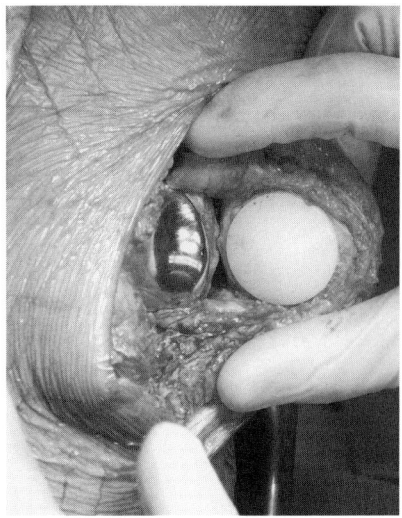

Fig. 9. Customized trochlear prosthesis and patellar prosthesis cemented in place.

Preoperative

1. The manufacturer's CT scanning protocol must be followed to ensure that bone geometry data are collected in the proper format and with sufficient resolution.
2. Because the posterior surface of the customized trochlear prosthesis is defined by CT scan data, any planned intraoperative osteophyte removal within the femoral trochlea must be communicated to the manufacturer before final prosthesis design. Removal of osteophytes is communicated readily through the customized bone model that is created for each case.
3. The strict indications and contraindications for patellofemoral arthroplasty must be respected. In the authors' experience, approximately 3% of patients undergoing knee arthroplasty are candidates for isolated patellofemoral arthroplasty.

Intraoperative

1. Residual problems with patellar alignment and tracking must be corrected at the time of surgery.
2. Only cartilage should be removed within the trochlear groove of the distal femur. The customized trochlear prosthesis is designed to rest against the subchondral bone of the trochlear groove. Unintentional removal of subchondral bone can compromise the fit of the customized trochlear prosthesis.
3. Patellofemoral joint overstuffing can be avoided by resecting more bone on the patellar side or by selecting a thinner patellar prosthesis.

Summary

The authors believe that the customized approach to patellofemoral arthroplasty effectively addresses the design deficiencies and difficulties in surgical technique associated with off-the-shelf trochlear prostheses. Progression of arthritic disease into the medial and lateral knee compartments often contributes to the need for patellofemoral prosthesis revision. Poorly fitting off-the-shelf prostheses can affect the mechanics of the knee joint (including the medial and lateral compartments) negatively, leading to disease progression into these compartments. The customized approach to patellofemoral arthroplasty is designed to restore the mechanics of the patellofemoral compartment and therefore maintain the native mechanics of the tibiofemoral compartments. Furthermore, the learning curve for customized patellofemoral arthroplasty is extremely short, because positioning and alignment of the customized trochlear prosthesis is determined preoperatively, thus eliminating intraoperative guesswork.

In the past few years, there has been a resurgence of interest in patellofemoral arthroplasty. Although the results of off-the-shelf patellofemoral prostheses have varied, the authors' results with a customized approach to patellofemoral arthroplasty are encouraging. The results of this customized approach demonstrate that it is a safe and effective treatment option for patients who have isolated patellofemoral arthritis.

References

[1] McAlindon TE, Snow S, Cooper C, et al. Radiographic patterns of osteoarthritis of the knee joint in the community: the importance of the patellofemoral joint. Ann Rheum Dis 1992;51(7):844–9.
[2] Lonner JH. Patellofemoral arthroplasty. J Am Acad Orthop Surg 2007;15(8):495–506.
[3] Mont MA, Haas S, Mullick T, et al. Total knee arthroplasty for patellofemoral arthritis. J Bone Joint Surg Am 2002;84:1977–81.
[4] Ackroyd CE, Chir B. Development and early results of a new patellofemoral arthroplasty. Clin Orthop Relat Res 2005;436:7–13.
[5] Arciero RA, Toomey HE. Patellofemoral arthroplasty. A three- to nine-year follow-up study. Clin Orthop Relat Res 1988;236:60–71.
[6] Argenson JN, Guillaume JM, Aubaniac JM. Is there a place for patellofemoral arthroplasty? Clin Orthop Relat Res 1995;321:162–7.
[7] Argenson JN, Flecher X, Parratte S, et al. Patellofemoral arthroplasty: an update. Clin Orthop Relat Res 2005;440:50–3.
[8] Blazina ME, Fox JM, Del Pizzo W, et al. Patellofemoral replacement. Clin Orthop Relat Res 1979;144:98–102.
[9] Cartier P, Sanouiller JL, Grelsamer R. Patellofemoral arthroplasty. 2- 12-year follow-up study. J Arthroplasty 1990;5:49–55.
[10] de Winter WE, Feith R, van Loon CJ. The Richards type II patellofemoral arthroplasty: 26 cases followed for 1–20 years. Acta Orthop Scand 2001;72:487–90.
[11] Kooijman HJ, Driessen AP, van Horn JR. Long-term results of patellofemoral arthroplasty. A report of 56 arthroplasties with 17 years of follow-up. J Bone Joint Surg Br 2003;85:836–40.
[12] Krajca-Radcliffe JB, Coker TP. Patellofemoral arthroplasty. A 2- to 18-year followup study. Clin Orthop Relat Res 1996;330:143–51.

[13] Lubinus HH. Patella glide bearing total replacement. Orthopedics 1979;2:119–27.
[14] Merchant AC. Early results with a total patellofemoral joint replacement arthroplasty prosthesis. J Arthroplasty 2004;19:829–36.
[15] Sisto DJ, Sarin VK. Custom patellofemoral arthroplasty of the knee. J Bone Joint Surg Am 2006;88(7):1475–80.
[16] Smith AM, Peckett WR, Butler-Manuel PA, et al. Treatment of patello-femoral arthritis using the Lubinus patello-femoral arthroplasty: a retrospective review. Knee 2002;9:27–30.
[17] Tauro B, Ackroyd CE, Newman JH, et al. The Lubinus patellofemoral arthroplasty. A five- to ten-year prospective study. J Bone Joint Surg Br 2001;83:696–701.
[18] Lonner JH. Patellofemoral arthroplasty: pros, cons, and design considerations. Clin Orthop Relat Res 2004;428:158–65.
[19] Fulkerson JP. Disorders of the patellofemoral joint. 4th edition. Philadelphia: Lippincott Williams & Wilkins; 2004.
[20] Leadbetter WB, Seyler TM, Ragland PS, et al. Indications, contraindications, and pitfalls of patellofemoral arthroplasty. J Bone Joint Surg Am 2006;88(Suppl 4):122–37.
[21] Ahlback S. Osteoarthrosis of the knee. A radiographic investigation. Acta Radiol Diagn (Stockh) 1968;277(Supp):7–72.
[22] Sisto DJ, Sarin VK. Custom patellofemoral arthroplasty of the knee: surgical technique. J Bone Joint Surg Am 2007;89(Suppl 2, Part 2):214–25.

Patellofemoral Arthroplasty in the Treatment of Patellofemoral Arthritis: Rationale and Outcomes in Younger Patients

Wayne B. Leadbetter, MD*

Center for Joint Preservation and Replacement, Rubin Institute for Advanced Orthopedics,
Sinai Hospital of Baltimore, 2401 West Belvedere Avenue, Baltimore, MD 21215, USA

Patellofemoral degenerative disease encompasses a spectrum of articular wear from severe chondrosis (Outerbridge III/IV with predominantly articular cartilage involvement) to advanced arthrosis (Outerbridge IV with exposed eburnated subchondral bone and remodeling). However, the Outerbridge classification technically refers to the morphologic stages of chondral injury or chondromalacia, whereas such classifications as the Kellgren-Lawrence are preferred to judge arthritis seen on plain radiographs [1,2]. Patellofemoral arthritis is often used as an encompassing term referring to all presentations of advanced articular wear [3]. Lesions may involve the patella facets, the trochlear groove, or both. The pathoetiology of excessive patellofemoral articular wear is multifactorial. In addition to trauma- and aging-related primary arthrosis, trochlear dysplasia is often a major contributing factor (Fig. 1) [4,5]. Patellofemoral malalignment associated with excessive lateral facet overload is a common precursor to articular degeneration [6]. The presence of patellofemoral instability or persistent femoral anteversion further complicates treatment [7]. The occurrence of any or a combination of these factors can lead to disabling patellofemoral pain even in young patients (age <45 years).

The present lack of efficacy or predictability of current surgical treatments for patellofemoral arthritis in any one individual has its roots in the problem of establishing the significant sources of the patient's presenting complaint, which is frequently nonspecific anterior knee pain [8]. In this sense, diagnosing patellofemoral arthritis as the source of "anterior knee pain syndrome" is analogous to diagnosing appendicitis as the cause of "acute abdominal pain." The key difference between symptomatic and asymptomatic patellofemoral arthritis is the amount of mechanical load transferred to the knee by physical activity [9]. There are few preoperative and essentially no validated intraoperative objective measurements available to determine the actual impact present operations have on such goals as extensor realignment or facet offloading [6,10]. Overcorrection and undercorrection errors are hard to avoid and probably occur more commonly than reported. This situation lends itself to a operative approach based somewhat on trial and error, where simplistic solutions are applied too early and aggressively, and more effective, but complex solutions are tried too late. Common recommended operations for the treatment of patellofemoral arthritis are, in roughly this order, chondroplasty, lateral release, soft tissue reconstruction, realignment or unloading osteotomy, biological articular restoration, and prosthetic resurfacing procedures. Many of these procedures require lengthy recovery with postoperative bracing or unweighting and can be associated with a legacy of technical and disuse complications, such as iatrogenic articular cartilage necrosis, quadriceps atrophy, arthrofibrosis, vastus lateralis insufficiency, osteotomy nonunion or fatigue fracture, and failed biological repair

---

No funding was received to support the research for or the preparation of this manuscript.
* 2646 Monocacy Ford Road, Frederick, MD 21701.
E-mail address: leadbettermd@aol.com

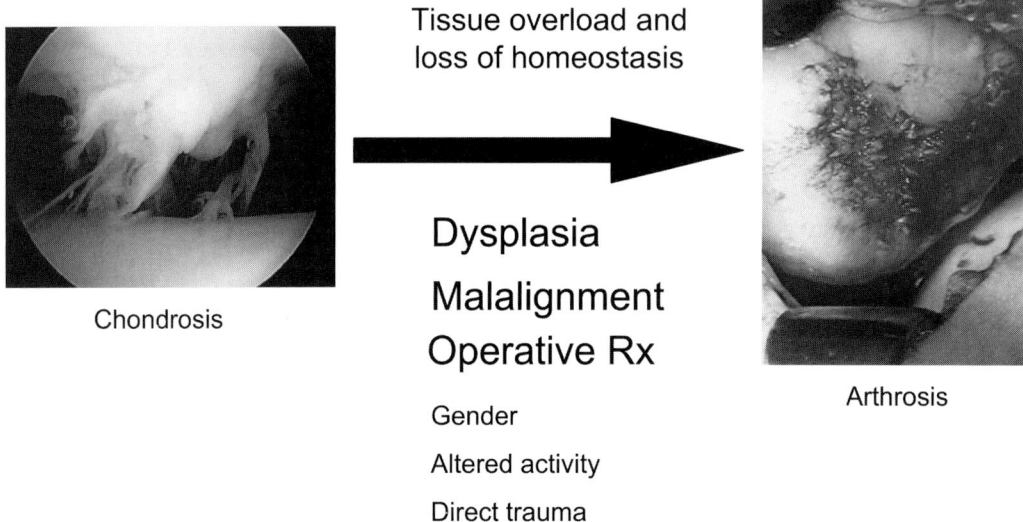

Fig. 1. Patellofemoral arthritis paradigm.

[11]. Thus, the end result of many of these well-intentioned surgical efforts can lead to an adverse outcome or "patella surgical cripple" instead of significant functional improvement [9]. The psychologic and economic toll of these outcomes on the patient cannot be underestimated.

The Avon patellofemoral arthroplasty (PFA) prosthesis (Stryker, Mahwah, New Jersey) was developed as a pragmatic response to more predictably address symptomatic isolated patellofemoral arthritic degeneration in a joint-conserving manner (Fig. 2) [12]. First used in older patients, isolated compartmental knee surgery offers significant potential advantages to the younger patient faced with disabling, degenerative patellofemoral pain when lengthy nonoperative treatments and previous surgical procedures have failed.

This article reviews pertinent aspects regarding the limitations of currently advocated operative interventions for patellofemoral degeneration. A literature review is provided of the reported experience with the Avon prosthesis as an alternative in select cases involving patients 45 years old or younger. Novel applications of this prosthesis are also discussed.

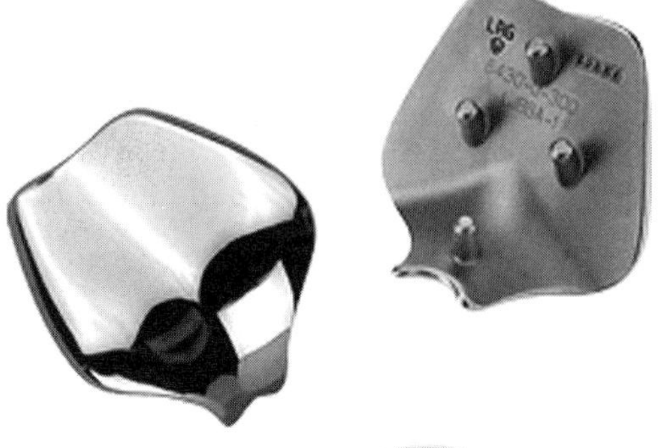

Limitations of current operative treatment of patellofemoral degenerative pain

Currently advocated operative treatments for advanced patellofemoral joint degeneration and arthritis remain controversial as to indications, patient selection, technique, and outcome reliability (Box 1) [3,13]. This problem of outcome reliability has long been appreciated [14]. Comments about the patellofemoral joint as "the forgotten joint," purgorative labeling of patellofemoral pain as the "low back pain" of the knee, and caveats that state "there are no heroes in patellofemoral surgery" reflect past pessimism about chances of success with surgical treatment [13].

To be successful, any operation must be directed at the correct dominant pathoeithiology.

Fig. 2. Avon patellofemoral prosthesis. (*Courtesy of* Stryker Orthopaedics, Mahwah, New Jersey; with permission.)

Box 1. Operative approaches for patellofemoral arthritis

Arthroscopic debridement
Microfracture articular restoration
Lateral release
Soft tissue realignment of the extensor mechanism
Anteromedialization tibial tubercle osteotomy
Mosiacplasty/autologous chondrocyte implantation
Lateral patella partial facetectomy
Patellectomy
Patellofemoral arthroplasty
Total knee arthroplasty

However, in patellofemoral arthritis, multiple factors often contribute to onset, progression, and disability. All these factors affect the patellofemoral joint via the promotion of excessive mechanical load (eg, malalignment) or deficient mechanical load (eg, atrophic) on the articular surfaces. Add to this challenge the observation that the patellofemoral joint is a hostile environment, especially for biological restoration. The joint is highly loaded, has minimal skeletal constraint, is functionally dependent on the integrity of muscle and soft tissue balance, is highly prone to dysplasia and congenital variation, and is dynamically influenced by limb skeletal alignment. Is it any wonder that no one operation will regularly solve any one particular patellar problem? Published series tend to be retrospective with short-term (<5 years) follow-up rarely achieving over 80% good results and even fewer excellent outcomes [15,16].

Aside from the temporary relief of degenerative related inflammatory events afforded by joint debridement, operative treatments attempt to relieve patellofemoral degenerative pain by successfully correcting the balance of forces on the patellofemoral joint by realignment, reducing articular surface overload by osteotomy, or increasing available joint surface contact, thereby decreasing load per unit area (ie, pressure), as with biological restoration or prosthetic resurfacing. The various options for operative salvage of patellofemoral joint degeneration are listed in Box 1.

Arthroscopic debridement with mechanical shavers or thermal devices continues to be a mainstay in the initial operative approach to patellofemoral chondral wear [17]. However, this approach invites significant concerns about the potential for iatrogenic thermal damage to healthy articular cartilage (Fig. 3) [18,19]. The use of such modalities is extremely technique-dependent [20]. Studies of diffuse patellar chondral debridement usually document modest short-term symptom and functional improvements, which are even less achievable in patients with patellofemoral malalignment and advanced grades of chondrosis [16]. The patellofemoral joint is not as responsive as the tibiofemoral joint to this form of treatment [15]. The real limitation of such isolated treatment is that it cannot address underlying promoting factors, such as biomechanical malalignment or dysplasia. Thus, as Teitge [21] has noted, "removal of articular

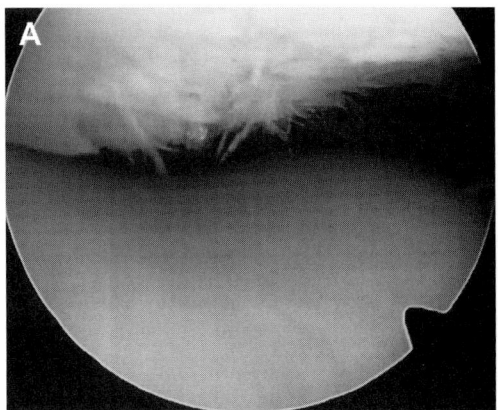 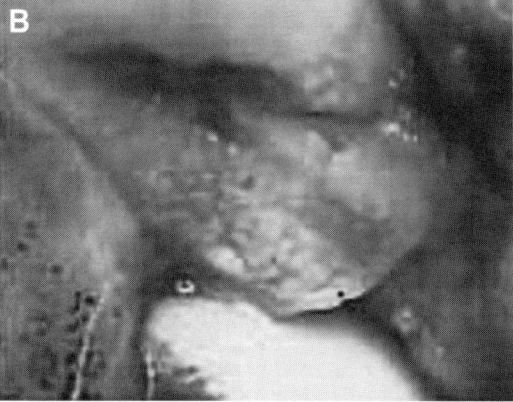

Fig. 3. (*A*) Arthroscopic image of 23-year-old female with grade III chondromalacia treated with thermal chondroplasty. (*B*) Same patient 1 year later showing grade IV erosion secondary to extensive thermal necrosis of patella. Patient proved to be unresponsive to an anteromedialization tibial tubercle osteotomy.

cartilage is tantamount to accelerating the rate of arthritic development." That said, most younger patients today with early stages of symptomatic patellofemoral degeneration (ie, chondromalacia patella) refractory to nonoperative management are initially offered a "conservative" arthroscopic procedure. To have any chance of success, the patient must continue to be compliant postoperatively with such measures as weight loss, behavior modification, and physical therapy as part of a comprehensive multimodal treatment program [22]. Furthermore, while a majority of patients with patellofemoral pain, moderate articular degeneration, or both may respond and deserve an initial attempt at nonoperative and palliative measures [8,22], in my experience there remains a significant number of patients who fall through the net of conventional care and evolve to intolerable patellofemoral-dominant disability.

Posttraumatic diffuse chondral damage treatment may not have as good a prognosis for isolated debridement [17]. When acute patellofemoral trauma results in complicated fracture or severe blunt force crush to the articular surfaces, the disability of extensive patellofemoral arthritis can ensue quickly, leaving few options other than patellectomy or arthroplasty. Patellectomy has fallen into disfavor because of unacceptable immediate problems with the recovery of extensor mechanism strength, gradual knee function deterioration, and potential compromise to the outcome of later total knee replacement [23]. In a series of 81 patients treated with patellectomy for isolated patellofemoral arthritis, Ackroyd and colleagues [24] achieved only a good result in 53%, a fair result in 26%, and a poor result in 21% of 87 knees at a mean follow-up of 6.5 years (range 2 to 22 years).

Anteromedialization tibial tubercle osteotomy (AMZ) has remained a mainstay in the treatment of patellofemoral articular degeneration since 1983 [25]. However, lesion location, extent, and patellofemoral alignment greatly influence outcome (Fig. 4) [14]. The operation is most effective in relieving pain in patients with bone-on-bone lateral facet arthritis with coincident lateral extensor mechanism malalignment [26]. This group achieved 87% good to excellent results. However, in all other lesion locations, the results drop off precipitously (55% to 20% good to excellent) [14]. Beck and colleagues [10] found that while AMZ may unload lateral trochlea lesions, the load effect upon the medial and central trochlea lesions is negligible or may increase. This may explain why anteromedialization in posttraumatic

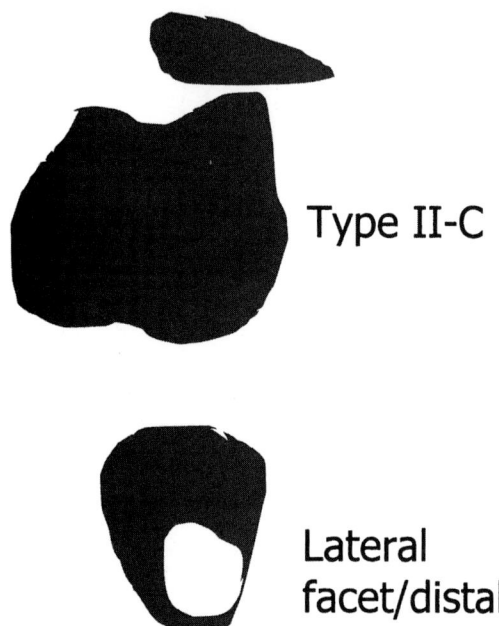

Fig. 4. Left knee Fulkerson-type IIC lateral patellofemoral malalignment with distal/lateral facet chondral lesion. This pattern is optimal for an AMZ procedure.

crush injuries do poorly [14]. Essentially, in a significant number of cases, AMZ results are not competitive with those achieved by modern PFA [27].

Partial lateral facetectomy can be useful in select patients with mild to moderate lateral extensor mechanism malalignment and isolated lateral patellofemoral arthritis. However, we agree with Yercan et al, that the procedure is much less reliable in severe malalignments and with medial or central patellofemoral lesions [28]. The procedure must include a lateral retinacular release, which must conserve the vastus lateralis muscle tendon. It is important to perform no more than a 1 to 1.5 cm resection of the lateral facet bone stock to avoid disturbing quadricepts function [28]. By conserving the remaining patellar bone, a PFA can still be used to salvage the 20% of failures reported with this approach [29].

Success with attempts at biological articular restoration in isolated patellofemoral arthritis has lagged behind success with femoral condyle lesions [30]. The results of patellofemoral articular restoration using osteochondral grafts (mosiacplasty) with either autogenous or fresh frozen allograft is not well documented, although such approaches in very young patients would seem reasonable. It has been useful primarily in trochlea lesions and rarely reported in the treatment of patella facet lesions, presumably because of the technical problems with dense recipient facet bone [31]. Nho and colleagues recently documented significant functional improvement using press-fit osteochondral autografts in 22 younger patients (mean age of 30 years old) with a mean follow-up of 28.7 months [32]. However, patients with patellofemoral malalignment did poorly; and MRI demonstrated a 30% failure of subchondral bone trabecular incorporation. There was no evidence of peripheral healing of the chondral plugs in any patient. Microfracture restoration is less helpful in the patellofemoral joint and requires a very specific rehabilitation, including bracing [33,34]. Such procedures can be technically demanding and costly. For example, biological restoration procedures, such as autologous cartilage implantation (ACI) require relatively lengthy protected recovery, can involve contentious authorization by insurers, and often demand large up-front prepayment risk by the hospital provider [35,36]. There is a paucity of literature documenting the outcome of ACI in the patellofemoral joint. Mandelbaum and colleagues [37] claimed short-term "apparent" improvement at 2 years with ACI treatment of trochlea defects (mean size 4.5 cm^2). Minas and Bryant [35] reported a 71% good to excellent result with patellofemoral ACI. However, while the lesions were extensive with a mean 4.86 cm^2 on the patella and 5.22 cm^2 on the trochlea, only four knees had both involved (ie, kissing) lesions. These were extensive procedures with 64% of patients requiring either tibial tubercle osteotomy or high tibial osteotomy to unload and protect the implantation. Biopsy analysis of graft tissue reveals that the morphology and genetic expression of the reparative tissue differs significantly from normal articular cartilage [38,39].

In summary, efforts to surgically treat the patellofemoral joint with present biological restoration techniques often appear compromised by the inherent hostile force–load milieux, the intrinsic limitations of healing in an avascular tissue, distortions of joint congruency, and lack of reliable constraints [21].

The argument against total knee arthroplasty and for patellofemoral arthroplasty

Admittedly, total knee arthroplasty (TKA) can achieve significant improvement in younger patients with severe tricompartmental arthritis [40–42]. Lonner and colleagues [43] reported a 91% good to excellent objective outcome in 32 knees in patients 40 years of age or younger with mean follow-up of 7.9 years. However, functional outcomes on the Knee Society Score were good to excellent in only 50% of patients. There is substantial evidence to question the reliability and validity of the Knee Society Score to assess the outcomes of either TKA or PFA [44]. Noble and colleagues [45] reported limitations in functional activities, such as moving laterally, turning, carrying loads, playing tennis, and gardening, in 52% of patients after TKR, compared with 22% in age-matched patients who had no reported knee complaints. Investigators concluded that normal aging effects could account for only about 40% of this deficit. As many as 7% to 19% of patients experience residual anterior knee pain when TKA is performed for isolated patellofemoral arthritis [46,47]. The residual detriment to knee joint kinematics, stability, and ligament balance caused by loss of the anterior cruciate ligament and the required bone resection in present day TKA has been documented [48]. Gait analysis in PFA has revealed correction of preoperative pathologic patterns that approach normal knee kinematics as well as improvement that is slightly better than that seen in TKA (Leadbetter, unpublished data, 2006). In older patients with isolated patellofemoral arthritis, the results of TKA have been reported as generally excellent with a range of 90% to 95% [46,47,49,50]. However, in these four papers, the average patient age was 70 years (range 47 to 88 years) and average follow-up was only 6.4 years (range, 3–11 years). Lateral release was required in 27% to 68% of knees. There was no assessment of specific recreational activity or significant quality of life limitations as previously mentioned by Noble and colleagues. More recently, Meding and colleagues [51] attempted to compare the outcome of TKA versus PFA in younger patients. The study consisted of a retrospective cohort of 27 patients (33 TKAs) with average follow-up of 6.2 years (range 2–12 years). The patients ranged in age from 38 to 60 years of age with a mean of 52 years. The investigators used comparative historical data on PFA outcomes in 10 studies [51]. Even though the results of TKA were only "as good…compared with younger patients undergoing patellofemoral arthroplasty," investigators concluded that TKA was the superior procedure. Without citing any extensive hands-on experience with PFA, the investigators nonetheless went on to make a sweeping indictment of PFA arthroplasty and labeled it an "ethically questionable" operation [51,52]. There were many disturbing aspects to these conclusions. Notable was the bias in the historical control. Of the 10 PFA papers reviewed, 6 involved first-generation patellofemoral designs that have either been abandoned or totally redesigned [53–57]. Meanwhile, 2 papers shared the same cohort only with longer follow-up [54,58]. It is claimed that reported revision rates for PFA ranged as high as 51% and that complications, or reoperations, or both ranged as high as 63% [51]. This is grossly misleading, as the reported results for revision and complications of current widely used PFAs (eg, Avon, Kinamed Custom PFA, and Low Contact Stress) are much more acceptable, ranging from 0% to 5% at a minimum 2-year follow-up [4,27,59,60]. Long-term results with PFA reflect the limitations of selective compartmental salvage. However, while Ackroyd and colleagues [27] noted a 20% radiologic progression of tibiofemoral arthritis at 5 years or greater with the Avon prosthesis, only 4% of knees required a revision operation at the time of follow-up. Cartier and colleagues [61] reported a survivorship of 75% at 6 to 10 years with the first-generation Richard I/II prosthesis. The need for revision was primarily tibiofemoral disease progression, uncorrected extensor malalignment, or technical error. Prosthetic loosening, wear, and infection were distinctly uncommon in contradistinction to some TKA experience [27,60,62]. In other words, an average of 75% to 80% of patients continued to enjoy the benefits of isolated patellofemoral resurfacing, while avoiding the technical, dysfunctional, and revision risks of present total knee arthroplasty. As of 2006, there have been 16 publications addressing PFA outcomes representing a total of 773 patients (912 knees) with an average age of 55.9 years (range 19 to 90 years), a mean follow-up of 5.7 years (range 0.16–24 years) with an average outcome of 88% improved function and pain relief (range 42%–96%).

The specter of the failed total knee replacement should not be downplayed. Revision rates for TKA have been correlated with younger age [63,64]. Typically, TKA reports do not stratify results for specific activities and sports. Mont and colleagues [65] surveyed tennis players (mean age 64 years) with TKA at a mean follow-up of 7 years and found high subjective satisfaction, but cautioned that the accumulative effect on prosthetic survivorship of many years of such high-performance activity has not been determined. One would assume that this cautionary advice would extend even more to a younger patient population. Yet, today more and more younger patients have high-performance expectations that are tacitly encouraged by prosthetic consumer marketing. Since we have seen no opinions that suggest that the recipient of a TKA at a younger age should be counseled not to expect at least one lifetime revision, the findings of Barrack and colleagues [66] regarding patient expectations after revision should be a concern to the surgeon. Generally, patients expected their replacement to last longer. More alarming was the finding that 66% disagreed with their surgeon as to the reason for failure and that only 69% were satisfied with their revision outcome [66]. Revised TKAs have been noted to have a consistent failure rate of 10% to 15% at 5 years [67]. Feinglass and colleagues [68] have noted that TKA revision rates are growing rapidly. This would suggest that the present comparative outcome standard of TKA durability to which PFA is being held is faulty. This means a large number of TKAs placed in younger patients can be expected to fail. In contradistinction, Lonner and colleagues [69] have noted that revision of the failed PFA does not compromise TKA outcome. There are no reported cases of any failed PFA requiring a knee fusion or eventual amputation. The estimated midterm accumulated failure rate for PFA has been calculated to be in the range of 20% to 25% [27,60,61]. However, Nicol and colleagues [70], in a review of 103 Avon PFA patients at mean follow-up of 7.1 years (range 5.5 to 8.5 years), found a revision rate of 14%. Radiographic disease progression was noted in only the medial compartment in just 7% of 89 patients in the same study who had not required revision to TKA at a mean follow-up of 4.6 years [70]. These results are comparable to reported midterm rates of failure of commonly advocated tibiofemoral unicompartmental arthroplasty, which range from 8% to 12% [71,72]. Not all progressive medial compartment disease is symptomatic (Fig. 5). PFA results remain very competitive with those of alternative procedures, such as unloading osteomy or cartilage transplantation, the results of which can also be diminished by progressive arthritic disease. Browne and colleagues [30] reported 5-year follow-up on 87 ACI patients, average age 37 years. There was a 30% failure rate. It was also noted that 70% of patients had already failed at least one prior attempted

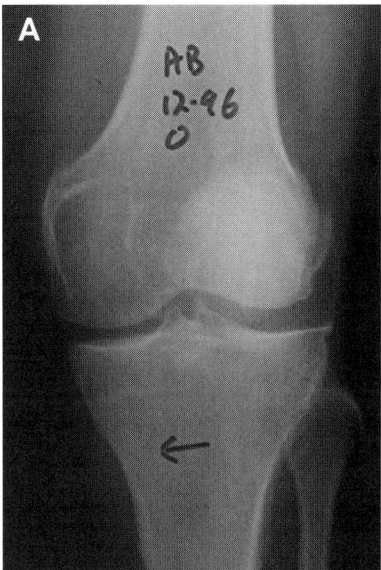 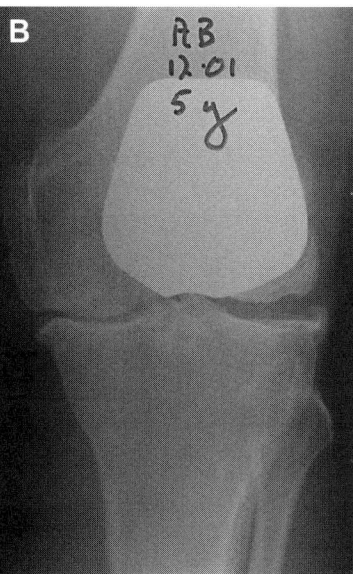

Fig. 5. Medial compartment arthritis progression post-Avon PFA. Patient remained functional and asymptomatic despite radiograph appearance. (*A*) Pre-op weightbearing plain AP radiograph left knee. Note normal medial compartment with Kellgren-Lawrence Stage I lateral change; (*B*) same patient five years post Avon PFA.Note Kellgren-Lawrence Stage III-IV radiologic arthritic progression medially and Stage III laterally. (*Courtesy of* C. Ackroyd.)

cartilage restoration. Fulkerson and colleagues [73] reported 75% good results and no excellent outcomes with AMZ when treating advanced patellofemoral arthritis.

Ultimately, the choice of PFA has its roots in evolving surgical thinking that places a greater priority on conserving native knee function and anatomy [48]. Technology is providing more options for the younger active patient in need of selective resurfacing for isolated knee arthritis. Compartmental salvage using modular and integrated devices is being employed with emphasis on resurfacing rather than replacement [48]. While it is recognized that present patellofemoral devices are not ideal, they offer a very reasonable midterm alternative for select patients. While weight remains a concern, many of our patients have been overweight with a body mass index (BMI) greater than 30. The PFA literature does not single out the obese patient as a poor candidate for PFA, but BMI levels in PFA have not been well reported. Specifically, no outcome studies have attributed an increase rate of PFA wear of prosthetic loosening to obesity. On the other hand, such patients typically do not make good candidates for unloading osteotomy or cartilage restoration. Because of frequent comorbidities, these patients often experience more operative complications after TKA procedures [74]. The effect of obesity on prosthetic survivorship and outcomes remains unclear [75,76], but it is safe to say that obese patients do not make inviting candidates for TKA.

Ultimately, I believe the current debate as to whether to choose a total knee arthroplasty or PFA for the treatment of patellofemoral degenerative disease has basically missed the point. The two operations have inherently different objectives, often involving a different subgroup of patients with significant differences in motive. TKA as reported today can lay claim to efficacy in relieving disability in patients over age 60 with isolated patellofemoral arthritis with reasonable hope of avoiding any further reoperations. TKA provides relief at least equal to PFA for advanced patellofemoral arthritic disease in patients younger than 60, but at a cost. The challenge is how to help patients who suffer from symptomatic patellofemoral articular wear at an age where the survivorship of their TKA would have to extend well over 30 years. Unfortunate patients in their 20s and 30s who fail repeated surgical interventions need a practical alternative to TKA for exactly the midterm improvement that can be achieved with patellofemoral arthroplasty. PFA has been documented to successfully address this challenge [4,59,60,77,78]. Forestalling the final solution of TKA in this group provides them the option of electing to wait for TKA technology to advance to a time when operative error is more controlled (eg, navigation), less bone resection is required, bearing surfaces improve even more, and cruxiate ligament function is routinely conserved.

Many younger patients fall into the expanded indication category for PFA of severe grade III/IV Outerbridge articular disease related to trochlear dyplasia, trauma, or correctible malalignment. The distribution of the lesions in such cases (eg, pantrochlear, panpatellar, or both) with chondropenia but minimal plain radiographic deterioration (ie, arthrosis) does not invite a TKA. The real prevalence of these cases is not well documented in the literature as the diagnosis of "isolated patellofemoral arthritis" is rarely stratified. However, all practicing orthopedic surgeons have experience with such failures, which often pose a crisis of choice in treatment. Based upon the previous discussion and my experience, neither surgeon nor patient is comfortable with the prospect of a TKA. Given an appropriate choice, patients invariably choose a PFA over a TKA and are willing to play the odds on durability versus risk, reserving a TKA as a backup. This is preferable to being told: "You are too young for a TKA. You'll just have to live with your problem." The issue is making available the choice. If the surgeon has but one hammer (ie, TKA) then the patient will be made that nail. While many arthroplasty and knee surgeons remain flexible on this issue [3,60,62], others are not [51].

Patellofemoral arthroplasty: experience in younger patients

The use of PFA in younger patients is not a new development. In the first report of successful PFA in 1979 by Blazina and colleagues [53], the average patient's age was 39 years with youngest recipient of a PFA being 19 years of age. As is typical, many of these patients had failed multiple operative procedures, particularly patelloplasty. Using a first-generation prosthesis (Richards I/II), 78% showed improved results at 1.8 years (range 0.7–3.5 years).

The results of the Avon PFA have been reviewed in younger patients [77,79]. This prosthesis was first introduced in Bristol, England, in 1996 and in the United States in 2001. Since that time the Avon has been widely adopted for its improved design and clinical outcomes [12,57]. Leadbetter and Ackroyd [77] presented the results of Avon PFA in 32 patients (42 knees) 45 years old or younger (mean age of 37 years, range 25–45 years) with a minimum 2-year follow-up. There were 28 women and 4 men. There was 3-year follow-up in 17 knees and over 5 years in 5 knees. Using outcome instruments that have been validated for patellofemoral disorders (ie, the Bristol Pain Score, the Bristol Movement Score, the Melbourne Patellar Score, and the Oxford Knee Score), 90.5% of patients achieved a good to excellent result with 95.6% prosthetic retention. There were no major complications or infections. Postoperative problems included residual pain or mechanical symptoms (9.5%), disease progression (7.1%) (see Fig. 5), persistent maltracking/subluxation (4.7%), patient selection error (eg, excessive preoperative flexion contracture) (2.3%) (Fig. 6), patellofemoral retinacular pain thought to be due to "overstuffing" (2.3%), and femoral component malrotation (2.3%). Although none of the previously cited reports of TKA for isolated patellofemoral arthritis mention the specific postoperative recreational activity, these young PFA patients resumed such pursuits as downhill skiing, ballet, cycling, hiking, manual labor, police work, tennis, and aerobic exercise. While it was stressed to the patients that such activities carry an unknown potential risk to longevity of their prosthesis, it remained their quality-of-life choice to engage in these activities. Given the option of wearing out a TKA as opposed to a PFA, it was their preference for the latter.

Clare and colleagues [78], reporting on 110 Avon PFA patients under the age of 55, found less predictable benefit when compared with a matched group of medial unicompartmental arthroplasty patients. This outcome is not entirely unexpected

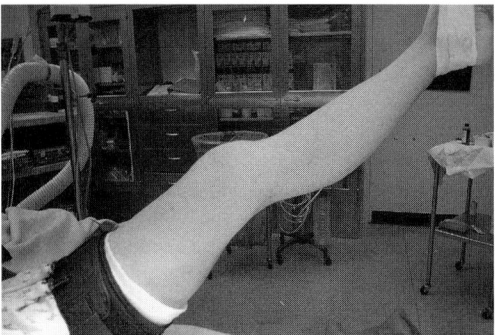

Fig. 6. Example of error in patient selection. Note preoperative flexion contracture. Patient failed to improve and required TKA. (*From* Leadbetter WB, Seyler TM, Ragland PS, et al. Indications, contraindications, and pitfalls of patellofemoral arthroplasty. J Bone Joint Surg Am 2006;88(Suppl 4):122–37; with permission.)

since advancing medial compartment wear is the most common unsolved late complication of PFA. Newer technology, such as the Journey Deuce (Smith and Nephew, London, United Kingdom), which resurfaces both patellofemoral and medial compartments, may improve future outcome [78]. The investigators further noted that patients with patellofemoral instability–related wear or trochlear dyplasia were generally helped [78].

What to consider when recommending or performing a patellofemoral arthroplasty

To be successful, a PFA operation must be predicated on accurate diagnosis, proper patient selection, suitable surgical technique, and appropriate prosthetic design [60,62,80]. The factors producing anterior and specifically patellofemoral arthritic pain are multiple; likewise the solutions.

Patients with symptomatic patellofemoral arthritis share a great overlap of conditions that could produce similar symptoms coincident with an abnormal patellofemoral plain roentgenogram. In contradistinction, patients under age 50 often present with relatively normal radiographs, but can have prominent patellofemoral pain and crepitation and are an even greater challenge to decision-making [8,9].

While much has been written about patient selection, not enough has been said about surgeon selection. The operating surgeon must be experienced or have acquired training with various options for patellofemoral realignment because a substantial proportion of patients with patellofemoral arthritis present with coincident extensor malalignment, or instability, or both. Competence with arthroplasty salvage and revision technique is implied by the variety of postoperative complications and failures. To avoid inappropriate use of PFA, the orthopedic surgeon must be familiar with the many nuances in the diagnostic evaluation of patellofemoral complaints [62]. This familiarity includes both soft tissue and osseous assessments [3]. Besides arthritis, a wide variety of conditions have been associated with the presence of patellofemoral pain, including transient synovitis, tendinopathy, quadriceps inhibition, patellofemoral instability or malalignment, activity-driven patellofemoral overload with loss of joint homeostasis, referred pain from the ipsilateral hip, discogenic pain, work- or litigation-motivated secondary gain, psychogenic pain or depression, chronic regional pain syndrome, and neuromata [7–9].

Box 2. Indications for patellofemoral arthroplasty

Degenerative osteoarthritis (ie, loss of joint space with osseous deformation) limited to the patellofemoral joint
Severe symptoms affecting daily activity referable to patellofemoral joint degeneration, unresponsive to lengthy (3–6 months) nonsurgical options, or failed prior conservative procedures (eg, lateral release, arthroscopic debridement, cartilage transplantation)
Posttraumatic osteoarthritis
Extensive grade III/IV chondrosis (ie, loss of joint space without osseous deformation of the patellofemoral joint space, particularly pantrochlear, medial facet, or proximal half of patella
Failed extensor unloading procedure (eg, Maquet, Fulkerson)
Patellofemoral malalignment/dysplasia–induced degeneration with or without instability

---

Box 3. Contraindications to patellofemoral arthroplasty

No attempt at nonoperative care or to rule out other sources of pain
Arthritis involving the tibiofemoral articulation greater than Kellgren grade I
Systemic inflammatory arthropathy
Osteoarthritis/chondrosis less than grade 3/4
Patella infera
Uncorrected patellofemoral instability/ malalignment
Uncorrected tibiofemoral mechanical malalignment (Q angle <177° or >183°)
Active infection
Evidence of chronic regional pain syndrome
Fixed-knee range-of-motion loss (minimum −10° extension; −110° flexion)
Psychogenic pain

Box 4. Additional factors that may adversely effect PFA outcome

Multiple antecedent procedures or extensive soft tissue trauma associated with residual quadriceps atrophy
History of prior arthrofibrosis
Ligamentous in the same joint or other operative site tibiofemoral instability
A postmenisectomy knee
Chondrocalcinosis
High patient activity or bent-knee use
Age under 40
Unrealistic patient expectations
A surgeon with lack of experience in arthroplasty or extensor mechanism realignment
Obesity (BMI >30)
Patella alta
Primary osteoarthritis
Male gender

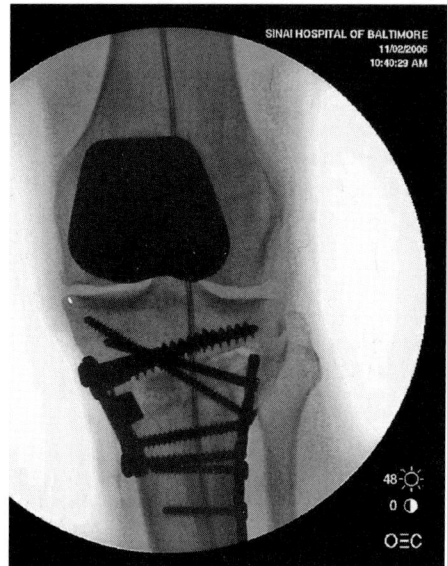

Fig. 7. Intraoperative image of a 46-year-old female who underwent Avon PFA 4 years previously. A high tibial osteotomy was performed for early medial compartment arthritis. Despite technical problems with the osteotomy (note additional lateral buttress plate to support lateral tibial cortex fracture), the patient did well and has avoided a TKA.

The indications and contraindications for PFA have been better defined in recent reviews (Boxes 2–4) [60,62]. Because tibiofemoral osteoarthritic progression is the most common postoperative

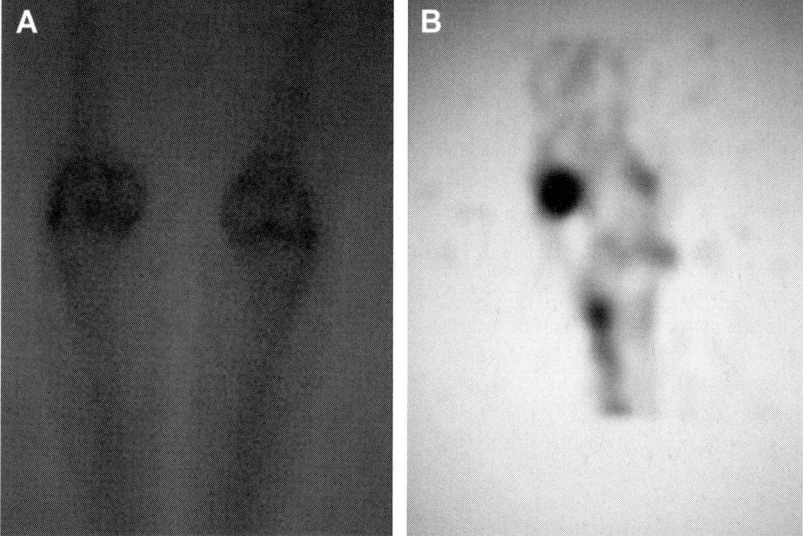

Fig. 8. (*A*) Preoperative standard technesium nucleotide bone scan of a patient with patellofemoral arthritis. (*B*) Same patient with a single photon emission CT augmentation of the same scan. Note heightened detail of uptake distribution concentrating in the patella. (*From* Leadbetter WB, Ragland PS, Mont MA. The appropriate use of patellofemoral arthroplasty: an analysis of reported indications, contraindications, and failures. Clin Orthop Relat Res 2005;436:91–9; with permission.)

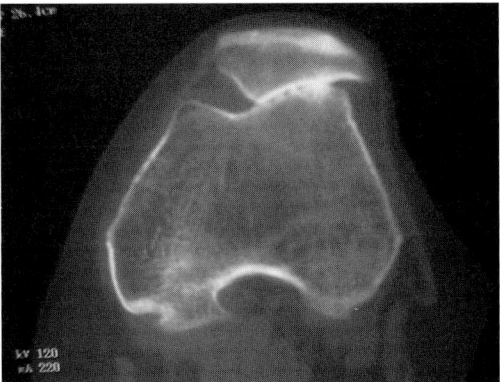

Fig. 9. Typical bony detail seen on axial CT scan of the arthritic patellofemoral joint. Pattern reveals the typical lateral dominant wear with moderate lateral malalignment.

problem with PFA, an extensive delineation of the medial and lateral compartments of the knee needs to be performed preoperatively to ascertain the degree of arthritis in other compartments. At a minimum, preoperative radiographs should include standing anteroposterior and lateral, Merchant, and 45° Rosenberg views. If there is concern as to axial leg malalignment, especially genu varum, a standing long leg film is required. Stress films to disclose ligamentous patholaxity may be useful. The surgeon needs to be wary of patients who do not have a near-neutral biomechanical axis. Such findings may need to be

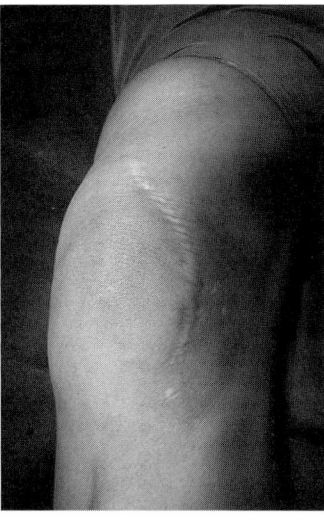

Fig. 11. Lateral incision from prior AMZ. Avoid wound complications by combining same skin incision with medial arthrotomy deep tissue approach.

addressed by other ancillary procedures, such as tibial osteotomies, to correct malalignment before performing a patellofemoral replacement. Because such malalignment corrections can require a large patient commitment when added to a PFA, a TKA is more likely to be more secure in older patients. However, we have been successful at avoiding TKA after PFA in early medical compartment disease progression by performing high tibial valgus osteotomy (Fig. 7). Radionuclide imaging can be helpful in isolating patellofemoral arthritic activity and pain [53]. In my experience,

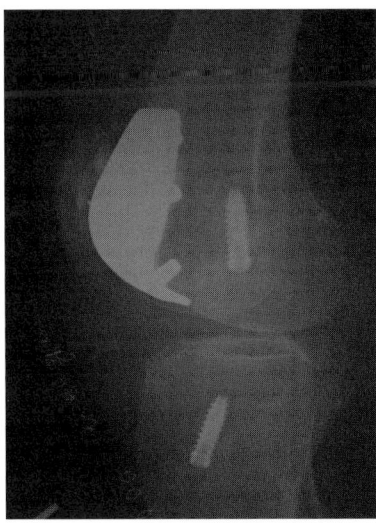

Fig. 10. Anterior cruciate ligament–deficient knee with isolated patellofemoral arthritis salvaged by staged anterior cruciate ligament reconstruction and PFA.

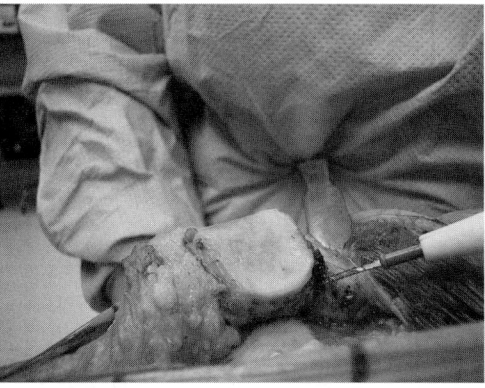

Fig. 12. Right knee intraoperative demonstration of the patella peel (periosteal lateral release). (*From* Leadbetter WB, Seyler TM, Ragland PS, et al. Indications, contraindications, and pitfalls of patellofemoral arthroplasty. J Bone Joint Surg Am 2006;88(Suppl 4):122–37; with permission.)

tomographic or spectrographic augmentation of such scans has improved accuracy of assessing compartmental sources of pain (Fig. 8). However, bone scan activity alone is not diagnostic of symptomatic patellofemoral arthritis [81]. More significance can be placed on bone scan activity once transient overuse or acute trauma has been excluded and after patient compliance with a proper patellofemoral-specific rehabilitative program. Scans are also useful in weeding out complex regional pain, which tends to present as a more global uptake. A negative scan can help exclude patellofemoral arthritis in psychogenic presentations or in cases involving secondary gain. If an adequate Merchant view cannot be reliably obtained, axial patellofemoral CT scans at 30°- 60°- 90° can provide useful information as to malalignment and joint-space loss (Fig. 9) [82]. MRI is helpful but less sensitive than knee arthroscopy in accurately assessing arthritic extent [83]. Used in combination, these tools provide reasonable assurance that a PFA may help relieve the patient's pain. Because almost all patients with symptomatic patellofemoral degeneration are offered at least one palliative arthroscopic procedure, disease extent and progress can be reasonably qualified. The anterior cruxiate–deficient knee is a relative contraindication to PFA. There is evidence that anteromedial rotatory knee pathoxlaxity can dynamically alter patellofemoral contact [84]. Reconstruction of the anterior cruciate ligament can be performed coincident with PFA (Fig. 10).

Surgical PFA technique can be challenging [80]. Fortunately, more reliable guide systems and better understanding of soft balancing of the extensor mechanism have evolved [78]. An incision that allows adequate exposure is the

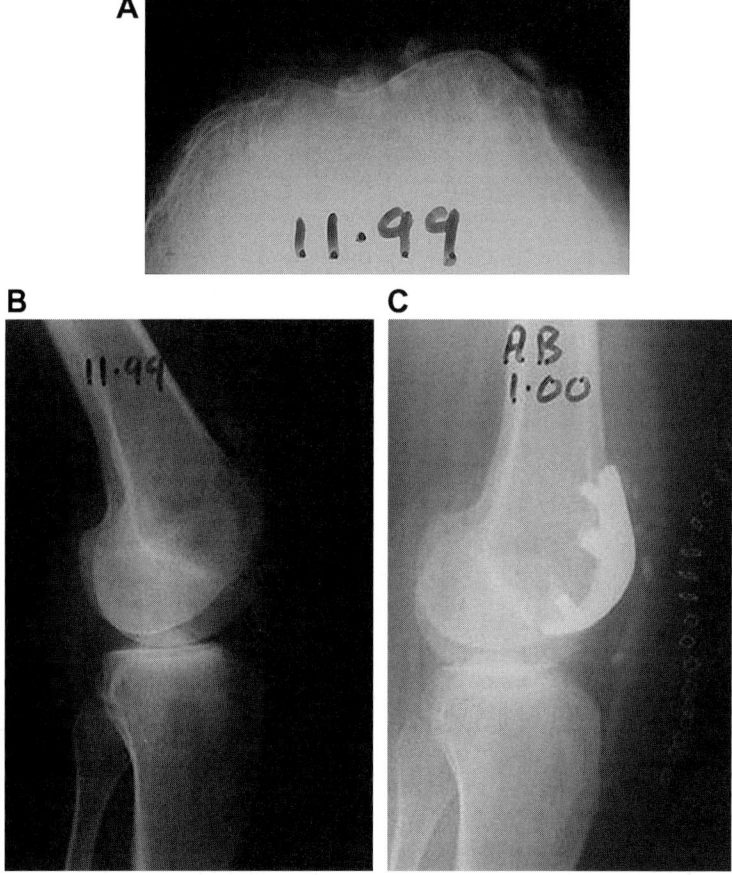

Fig. 13. (*A, B*) Preoperative plain radiographs of previously patellectomized patient treated with PFA and soft tissue extensor realignment for chronic extensor subluxation. (*C*) Post-operative appearance after Avon PFA used to improve trochlear constraint and reduce pain. (*Courtesy of* C. Ackroyd.)

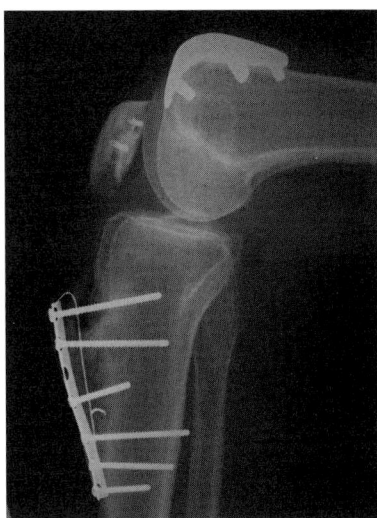

Fig. 14. Forty-five-year-old female 9 years post-AMZ with complications, 7 years post-Avon PFA salvage. Patient remains highly functional despite patella infera from repeated scarring. (*From* Leadbetter WB, Ragland PS, Mont MA. The appropriate use of patellofemoral arthroplasty: an analysis of reported indications, contraindications, and failures. Clin Orthop Relat Res 2005;436:91–9; with permission.)

correct one. This may vary with the circumstances of the patient. It is often possible and, in my opinion, desirable to conserve a portion of the vastus medialis obliqus (VMO) attachment, especially because most of these patients present with quadriceps dysfunction due to pain inhibition and disuse. Conserving some attachment of the VMO helps maintain an important dynamic medial force vector on the patella postoperatively. Therefore, in most cases, we have not had to resort to a full paramedian incision. If exposure is compromised, then one can simply extend the vastus release proximally (what I refer to as a vastus medialis "snip") until lateral translation and eversion of the patella is possible. No deliberate attempt is made to imitate a pure minimal incisional approach. However, with experience, the surgeon can easily reduce the extent of soft tissue disruptions that can retard recovery [78]. In patients who present with a prior Fulkerson-type realignment and large lateral incision, I recommend the use of the same lateral incision to avoid wound-healing problems (Fig. 11). The deep approach to the joint can then proceed paramedially, again conserving the VMO as much as possible. Place the femoral prosthesis in slight external rotation using the transepicondylar axis to avoid tightening the lateral retinaculum in flexion and to discourage patella subluxation. Prepare the patella resection carefully with pre- and post-resection measurement to leave at least 10-mm residual thickness. I prefer an instrumented resection rather than free hand. One difference between the PFA and the TKA techniques is not readily apparent. Namely, in flexion, medialization of the patella prosthesis

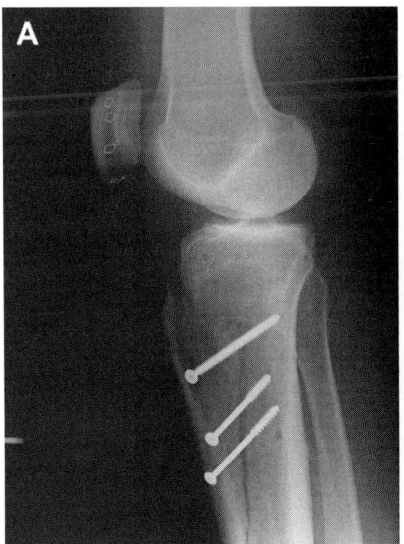 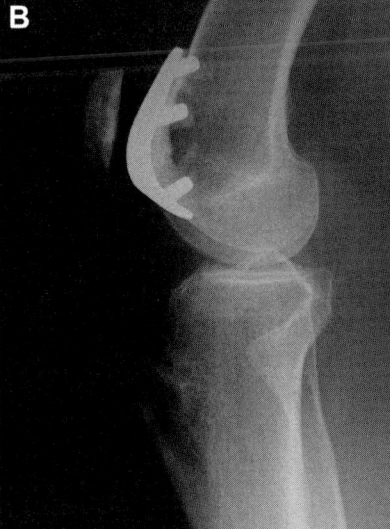

Fig. 15. (*A*) Same patient as in Fig. 3 post–Fulkerson osteotomy. (*B*) Same patient after Avon PFA salvage of failed AMZ.

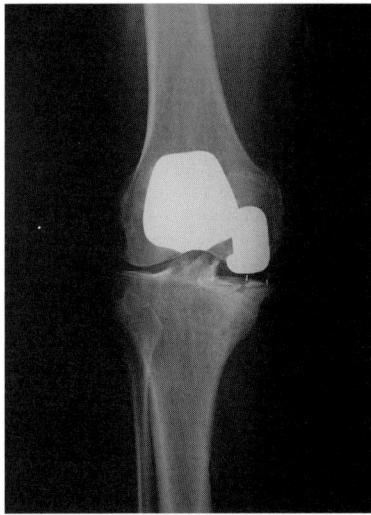

Fig. 16. Combined Avon PFA and medial unicompartment salvage.

encourages impingement on the medial femoral condyle in knee flexion. Place the patella component slightly less medial as long as tracking is not adversely affected. Finally, because soft tissue balancing is critical to stability, I routinely perform a "patellar retinacular peel" as described by Shaw (Fig. 12) [85]. This technique is useful in both TKA and PFA to avoid a formal lateral patellar release, which can further destabilize patella tracking as well as add morbidity. I have found the lateral patella chamfer cut to be useful to avoid lateral facet osteophytic impingement on the femur and allow further decompression to the lateral retinaculum as well [86]. More extensive discussion of PFA technique can be found in the literature [59,60,80].

Prosthetic design has been correlated with surgical success. At one point, the Lubinus prosthesis accounted for 27.9% of reported PFA failures [62]. These failures were linked to the lack of adaptability of the femoral component and led to its abandonment [57,87]. Lonner [57] has delineated the features of more successful prosthetic design. The Avon prosthesis is typical of the second-generation designs that incorporate better sizing; a more-forgiving, less-constrained femoral flange for patella capture; and a lower lateral profile with a radius of curvature that better fits the femoral groove [12]. When severe patellofemoral dysplasia is encountered, a custom prosthesis may be the best choice [4]. Newer PFA prostheses are providing more elaborate guide systems to help avoid operative error [78].

Novel applications of patellofemoral arthroplasty

PFA can be useful in some difficult clinical situations. Ackroyd and colleagues [88] have described salvage of the persistently painful knee with extensor subluxation after patellectomy. In three patients, the trochlear portion of the

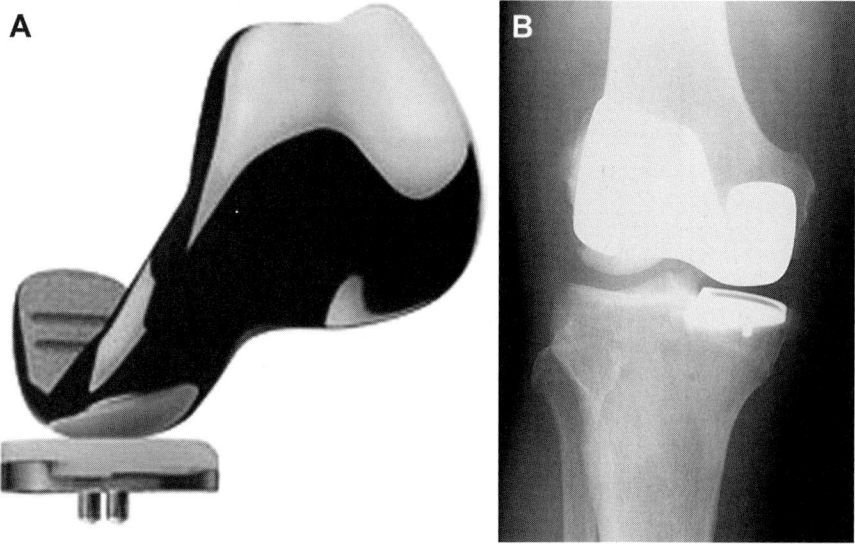

Fig. 17. (A) Model of the Journey Deuce bicompartmental prosthesis. (B) Radiographic appearance of the same implant. (A *courtesy of* Smith & Nephew Orthopedic Division, Memphis, Tennessee.)

Avon prosthesis was used to increase trochlear constraint (Fig. 13).

We have been moderately successful with salvage of the failed Fulkerson osteotomy with persistent arthritic pain. Of nine case results, seven were rated objectively good and two fair. The longest follow-up has been in a woman who experienced fracture complications with nonunion of her original osteotomy at age 36 (Fig. 14). Despite the presence of patella infera, she still functions at age 45 at a high level and has bilateral PFAs. The youngest such patient presented at 23 years of age with progressive patellofemoral degeneration due to dysplasia and malalignment. She also represented a case of iatragenic chondral injury secondary to thermal patella chondroplasty (see Fig. 3). Despite multiple strategies, including attempts at extensor realignment and tibial tubercle osteotomy, she required bilateral prosthetic salvage (Fig. 15). She has had immediate functional improvement, with no significant residual symptoms. Interestingly, all PFA patients preferred their PFA recovery to their osteotomy experience. All were off crutch support within 2 to 3 weeks.

Finally, PFA has been employed as a combined salvage with both medial unicompartmental arthroplasty (Fig. 16) [89] and with ACI cartilage restoration [90].

Summary

PFA is a re-emerging technology that has earned its place in the lexicon of patellofemoral treatment by long-established experience and continuing efforts at refinement. PFA has proven to have versatile applications. With improvements in our ability to radiologically detect the presence and predict the progression of osteoarthritis and cartilage degeneration, we will become more successful in compartmental salvage of knee arthritis. New developments in MRI hold that promise [91]. New bicompartmental prosthetic designs are now available to improve PFA survival while conserving the cruxiate ligaments (Fig. 17). In younger patients, PFA is a reasonable choice in select cases to extend function and reduce pain while avoiding a more complex TKA. While the argument has been made that TKA is the procedure of choice in these patients, I would submit that in the hands of the low-volume orthopedic surgeon such treatment is more likely to fail than a PFA [64]. PFA is not a panacea and certainly requires its own subset of surgical abilities, not the least of which is conservative judgment and a genuine interest in patellofemoral pain disorders. Like unicompartment knee arthroplasty, it remains an intermediate solution for some patients. Because no current surgical intervention can attain a normal knee, PFA remains an important option.

References

[1] Outerbridge RE. The etiology of chondromalacia patellae. J Bone Joint Surg Br 1961;43:752–7.

[2] Kellgren JH, Lawrence JS. Radiological assessment of osteo-arthrosis. Ann Rheum Dis 1957;16(4): 494–502.

[3] Saleh KJ, Arendt EA, Eldridge J, et al. Symposium. Operative treatment of patellofemoral arthritis. 10.2106/JBJS.D.03035. J Bone Joint Surg Am 2005; 87(3):659–71.

[4] Sisto DJ, Sarin VK. Custom patellofemoral arthroplasty of the knee. J Bone Joint Surg Am 2006; 88(7):1475–80.

[5] Dejour H, Walch HG, Neyret P, et al. [Dysplasia of the femoral trochlea]. Rev Chir Orthop Reparatrice Appar Mot 1990;76(1):45–54 [in French].

[6] Arendt E. Anatomy and malalignment of the patellofemoral joint: its relation to patellofemoral arthrosis. Clin Orthop Relat Res 2005;436:71–5.

[7] Post WR, Teitge R, Amis A. Patellofemoral malalignment: looking beyond the viewbox. Clin Sports Med 2002;21(3):521–46, x.

[8] Post WR. Anterior knee pain: diagnosis and treatment. J Am Acad Orthop Surg 2005;13(8):534–43.

[9] Dye SF. The pathophysiology of patellofemoral pain: a tissue homeostasis perspective. Clin Orthop Relat Res 2005;436:100–10.

[10] Beck PR, Thomas AL, Farr J, et al. Trochlear contact pressures after anteromedialization of the tibial tubercle. Am J Sports Med 2005;33(11):1710–5.

[11] Hillsgroove Dc PL. The patella. In: Scuderi GR, editor. The patella. New York: Springer-Verlag; 1995. p. 277–90.

[12] Ackroyd CE, Chir B. Development and early results of a new patellofemoral arthroplasty. Clin Orthop Relat Res 2005;436:7–13.

[13] Mihalko WM, Boachie-Adjei Y, Spang JT, et al. Controversies and techniques in the surgical management of patellofemoral arthritis. J Bone Joint Surg Am 2007;89:2788–802.

[14] Pidoriano AJ, Weinstein RN, Buuck DA, et al. Correlation of patellar articular lesions with results from anteromedial tibial tubercle transfer. Am J Sports Med 1997;25(4):533–7.

[15] Voloshin I, Morse KR, Alfred CD, et al. Arthroscopic evaluation of radiofrequency chondroplasty of the knee. Am J Sports Med 2007;35(10): 1702–7.

[16] Herrenbruck Tm MD, Parker RD. Operative management of patellofemoral pain with degenerative arthritis. Sports Med Arthrosc 2001;9(4):312–24.

[17] Federico DJ, Reider B. Results of isolated patellar debridement for patellofemoral pain in patients with normal patellar alignment. Am J Sports Med 1997;25(5):663–9.

[18] Caffey S, McPherson E, Moore B, et al. Effects of radiofrequency energy on human articular cartilage: an analysis of 5 systems. Am J Sports Med 2005;33(7):1035–9.

[19] Bonutti PM, Seyler TM, Delanois RE, et al. Osteonecrosis of the knee after laser or radiofrequency-assisted arthroscopy: treatment with minimally invasive knee arthroplasty. J Bone Joint Surg Am 2006;88(Suppl 3):69–75.

[20] Is there a role for radiofrequency-based ablation in the treatment of chondral lesions? [review]. Am J Orthop 2005;34(Suppl 8):3–15.

[21] Teitge R. Treatment of complications of patellofemoral surgery. Oper Tech Sports Med 1994;2(4):317–34.

[22] Kalenak A. Nonoperative treatment of patellofemoral disorders. Sports Med Arthrosc 1994;2(3):237–42.

[23] Paletta GA Jr, Laskin RS. Total knee arthroplasty after a previous patellectomy. J Bone Joint Surg Am 1995;77(11):1708–12.

[24] Ackroyd CE, Polyzoides AJ. Patellectomy for osteoarthritis. A study of eighty-one patients followed from two to twenty-two years. J Bone Joint Surg Br 1978;60-B(3):353–7.

[25] Fulkerson JP. Anteromedialization of the tibial tuberosity for patellofemoral malalignment. Clin Orthop Relat Res 1983;177:176–81.

[26] Farr J, Schepsis A, Cole B, et al. Anteromedialization: review and technique. J Knee Surg 2007;20(2):120–8.

[27] Ackroyd CE, Newman JH, Evans R, et al. The Avon patellofemoral arthroplasty: five-year survivorship and functional results. J Bone Joint Surg Br 2007;89(3):310–5.

[28] Yercan HS, Ait Si Selmi T, Neyret P. The treatment of patellofemoral osteoarthritis with partial lateral facetectomy. Clin Orthop Relat Res 2005;436:14–9.

[29] Paulos PE, O'Connor DL, Karistinos A. Partial lateral patellar facetectomy for treatment of arthritis due to lateral patellar compression syndrome. J Arthrscopic and Rel Surg 2008;24:547–53.

[30] Browne JE, Anderson AF, Arciero R, et al. Clinical outcome of autologous chondrocyte implantation at 5 years in US subjects. Clin Orthop Relat Res 2005;436:237–45.

[31] Torga Spak R, Teitge RA. Fresh osteochondral allografts for patellofemoral arthritis: long-term follow up. Clin Orthop Relat Res 2006;444:193–200.

[32] Nho SJ, Foo LF, Green DM, et al. Magnetic resonance imaging and clinical evaluation of patellar resurfacing with press-fit osteochondral autograft plugs. Am J Sports Med 2008;36(6):1101–9.

[33] Yen YM, Cascio B, O'Brien L, et al. Treatment of osteoarthritis of the knee with microfracture and rehabilitation. Med Sci Sports Exerc 2008;40(2):200–5.

[34] Riegger-Krugh CL, McCarty EC, Robinson MS, et al. Autologous chondrocyte implantation: current surgery and rehabilitation. Med Sci Sports Exerc 2008;40(2):206–14.

[35] Minas T, Bryant T. The role of autologous chondrocyte implantation in the patellofemoral joint. Clin Orthop Relat Res 2005;436:30–9.

[36] Knutsen G, Drogset JO, Engebretsen L, et al. A randomized trial comparing autologous chondrocyte implantation with microfracture. Findings at five years. J Bone Joint Surg Am 2007;89(10):2105–12.

[37] Mandelbaum B, Browne JE, Fu F, et al. Treatment outcomes of autologous chondrocyte implantation for full-thickness articular cartilage defects of the trochlea. Am J Sports Med 2007;35(6):915–21.

[38] Grigolo B, Roseti L, De Franceschi L, et al. Molecular and immunohistological characterization of human cartilage two years following autologous cell transplantation. J Bone Joint Surg Am 2005;87(1):46–57.

[39] LaPrade RF, Bursch LS, Olson EJ, et al. Histologic and immunohistochemical characteristics of failed articular cartilage resurfacing procedures for osteochondritis of the knee: a case series. Am J Sports Med 2008;36(2):360–8.

[40] Whiteside LA, Vigano R. Young and heavy patients with a cementless TKA do as well as older and lightweight patients. Clin Orthop Relat Res 2007;464:93–8.

[41] Duffy GP, Trousdale RT, Stuart MJ. Total knee arthroplasty in patients 55 years old or younger. 10- to 17-year results. Clin Orthop Relat Res 1998;356:22–7.

[42] Mont MA, Lee CW, Sheldon M, et al. Total knee arthroplasty in patients ≤ 50 years old. J Arthroplasty 2002;17(5):538–43.

[43] Lonner JH, Hershman S, Mont M, et al. Total knee arthroplasty in patients 40 years of age and younger with osteoarthritis. Clin Orthop Relat Res 2000;380:85–90.

[44] Paxton EW, Fithian DC. Outcome instruments for patellofemoral arthroplasty. Clin Orthop Relat Res 2005;436:66–70.

[45] Noble PC, Gordon MJ, Weiss JM, et al. Does total knee replacement restore normal knee function? Clin Orthop Relat Res 2005;431:157–65.

[46] Mont MA, Haas S, Mullick T, et al. Total knee arthroplasty for patellofemoral arthritis. J Bone Joint Surg Am 2002;84(11):1977–81.

[47] Parvizi J, Stuart MJ, Pagnano MW, et al. Total knee arthroplasty in patients with isolated patellofemoral arthritis. Clin Orthop Relat Res 2001;392:147–52.

[48] Engh GA. Advances in knee arthroplasty for younger patients: traditional knee arthroplasty is prologue, the future for knee arthroplasty is prescient. Orthopedics 2007;30(Suppl 8):55–7.

[49] Laskin RS, van Steijn M. Total knee replacement for patients with patellofemoral arthritis. Clin Orthop Relat Res 1999;367:89–95.
[50] Dalury DF. Total knee replacement for patellofemoral disease. J Knee Surg 2005;18(4):274–7.
[51] Meding JB, Wing JT, Keating EM, et al. Total knee arthroplasty for isolated patellofemoral arthritis in younger patients. Clin Orthop Relat Res 2007;464: 78–82.
[52] Keating EM, Meding JB, Faris PM, et al. Long-term followup of nonmodular total knee replacements. Clin Orthop Relat Res 2002;404:34–9.
[53] Blazina ME, Fox JM, Del Pizzo W, et al. Patellofemoral replacement. Clin Orthop Relat Res 1979;144: 98–102.
[54] Argenson JN, Guillaume JM, Aubaniac JM. Is there a place for patellofemoral arthroplasty? Clin Orthop Relat Res 1995;321:162–7.
[55] deWinter We FR, van Loon CJ. The Richards type II patellofemoral arthroplasty: 26 cases followed for 1–20 years. Acta Orthop Scand 2001;72:487–90.
[56] Kooijman HJ, Driessen AP, van Horn JR. Long-term results of patellofemoral arthroplasty. A report of 56 arthroplasties with 17 years of follow-up. J Bone Joint Surg Br 2003;85(6):836–40.
[57] Lonner JH. Patellofemoral arthroplasty: pros, cons, and design considerations. Clin Orthop Relat Res 2004;428:158–65.
[58] Argenson JN, Flecher X, Parratte S, et al. Patellofemoral arthroplasty: an update. Clin Orthop Relat Res 2005;440:50–3.
[59] Merchant AC. A modular prosthesis for patellofemoral arthroplasty: design and initial results. Clin Orthop Relat Res 2005;436:40–6.
[60] Lonner JH. Patellofemoral arthroplasty. J Am Acad Orthop Surg 2007;15(8):495–506.
[61] Cartier P, Sanouiller JL, Khefacha A. Long-term results with the first patellofemoral prosthesis. Clin Orthop Relat Res 2005;436:47–54.
[62] Leadbetter WB, Ragland PS, Mont MA. The appropriate use of patellofemoral arthroplasty: an analysis of reported indications, contraindications, and failures. Clin Orthop Relat Res 2005;436:91–9.
[63] Harrysson OL, Robertsson O, Nayfeh JF. Higher cumulative revision rate of knee arthroplasties in younger patients with osteoarthritis. Clin Orthop Relat Res 2004;421:162–8.
[64] Heck DA, Melfi CA, Mamlin LA, et al. Revision rates after knee replacement in the United States. Med Care 1998;36(5):661–9.
[65] Mont MA, Rajadhyaksha AD, Marxen JL, et al. Tennis after total knee arthroplasty. Am J Sports Med 2002;30(2):163–6.
[66] Barrack RL, Skinner HB, Cook SD, et al. Revision total knee arthroplasty: the patient's perspective. Clin Orthop Relat Res 2007;464:146–50.
[67] Sierra Rj PM, Trusdale RT. Abstract: reoperations after 3200 revision TKRs: rate, etiology, and lessons learned. In 70th Annual Meeting Proceedings. Rosemont (IL): American Academy of Orthopaedic Surgeons 2003. p. 574.
[68] Feinglass J, Koo S, Koh J. Revision total knee arthroplasty complication rates in Northern Illinois. Clin Orthop Relat Res 2004;429:279–85.
[69] Lonner JH, Jasko JG, Booth RE Jr. Revision of a failed patellofemoral arthroplasty to a total knee arthroplasty. J Bone Joint Surg Am 2006;88(11): 2337–42.
[70] Nicol SG, Loveridge JM, Weale AE, et al. Arthritis progression after patellofemoral joint replacement. Knee 2006;13(4):290–5.
[71] Cartier P, Khefacha A, Sanouiller JL, et al. Unicondylar knee arthroplasty in middle-aged patients: a minimum 5-year follow-up. Orthopedics 2007; 30(Suppl 8):62–5.
[72] Swienckowski JJ, Pennington DW. Unicompartmental knee arthroplasty in patients sixty years of age or younger. J Bone Joint Surg Am 2004; 86(Suppl 1 Pt 2):131–42.
[73] Fulkerson JP, Becker GJ, Meaney JA, et al. Anteromedial tibial tubercle transfer without bone graft. Am J Sports Med 1990;18(5):490–6 [discussion: 496–7].
[74] Miric A, Lim M, Kahn B, et al. Perioperative morbidity following total knee arthroplasty among obese patients. J Knee Surg 2002;15(2):77–83.
[75] Mont MA, Mathur SK, Krackow KA, et al. Cementless total knee arthroplasty in obese patients. A comparison with a matched control group. J Arthroplasty 1996;11(2):153–6.
[76] Nicol SG, Loveridge JM, Weale AE, et al. Arthritis progression after patellofemoral joint replacement. Knee 2006;13(4):290–5.
[77] Leadbetter WB, Ackroyd CE. Patellofemoral arthroplasty results in young patients (<45 years). Proceedings of the Annual Meeting of the American Academy of Orthopaedic Surgeons. American Academy of Orthopaedic Surgery. San Diego, 2007.
[78] Newman JH. Patellofemoral arthritis and its management with isolated patellofemoral replacement: a personal experience. Orthopedics 2007;30(Suppl 8): 58–61.
[79] Clare TD NJ, Ackroyd CE, Evans R. Early results in 100 cases of patello-femoral replacement in patients under 55 years of age. Proceedings of ESSKA Innsbrook, 2006.
[80] Leadbetter WB, Seyler TM, Ragland PS, et al. Indications, contraindications, and pitfalls of patellofemoral arthroplasty. J Bone Joint Surg Am 2006; 88(Suppl 4):122–37.
[81] Dye SF, Boll DA. Radionuclide imaging of the patellofemoral joint in young adults with anterior knee pain. Orthop Clin North Am 1986;17(2): 249–62.
[82] Schutzer SF, Ramsby GR, Fulkerson JP. Computed tomographic classification of patellofemoral pain patients. Orthop Clin North Am 1986;17(2): 235–48.

[83] Kuikka PI, Kiuru MJ, Niva MH, et al. Sensitivity of routine 1.0-Tesla magnetic resonance imaging versus arthroscopy as gold standard in fresh traumatic chondral lesions of the knee in young adults. Arthroscopy 2006;22(10):1033–9.

[84] Hsieh YF, Draganich LF, Ho SH, et al. The effects of removal and reconstruction of the anterior cruciate ligament on the contact characteristics of the patellofemoral joint. Am J Sports Med 2002;30(1):121–7.

[85] Shaw JA. Patellar retinacular peel: an alternative to lateral retinacular release in total knee arthroplasty. Am J Orthop 2003;32(4):189–92.

[86] Lonner JH. Lateral patellar chamfer in total knee arthroplasty. Am J Orthop 2001;30(9):713–4.

[87] Tauro B, Ackroyd CE, Newman JH, et al. The Lubinus patellofemoral arthroplasty. A five- to ten-year prospective study. J Bone Joint Surg Br 2001;83(5):696–701.

[88] Ackroyd CE, Smith EJ, Newman JH. Trochlear resurfacing for extensor mechanism instability following patellectomy. Knee 2004;11(2):109–11.

[89] Antoniou J, Hadjipavlou A, Enker P, et al. Unicompartmental knee arthroplasty with patelloplasty. Int Orthop 1996;20(2):94–9.

[90] Lonner JH, Mehta S, Booth RE Jr. Ipsilateral patellofemoral arthroplasty and autogenous osteochondral femoral condylar transplantation. J Arthroplasty 2007;22(8):1130–6.

[91] Burstein D, GM. New MRI techniques for imaging cartilage. International Society of Arthroscopy, Knee Surgery, and Orthopaedic Sports Medicine Newsletter 2002;2:14–6.

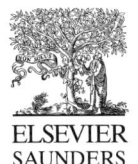

Results of Total Knee Replacement for Isolated Patellofemoral Arthritis: When Not to Perform a Patellofemoral Arthroplasty

Ronald E. Delanois, MD[a], Mike S. McGrath, MD[a], Slif D. Ulrich, MD[a], David R. Marker, BS[a], Thorsten M. Seyler, MD[a], Peter M. Bonutti, MD[b], Michael A. Mont, MD[a],*

[a]Center for Joint Preservation and Reconstruction, Rubin Institute for Advanced Orthopedics, Sinai Hospital of Baltimore, 2401 West Belvedere Avenue, Baltimore, MD 21215, USA
[b]Bonutti Clinic, 1303 West Evergreen Avenue, Effingham, IL 62401, USA

Isolated patellofemoral arthritis is found in 5% to 10% of patients who present to physicians for diagnosis or treatment of knee pain [1]. It is present in up to 15% of patients who are older than 60 years [2]. Causes of this condition include prior trauma to the patella, malalignment of the patellofemoral joint, congenital trochlear dysplasia, and degeneration secondary to age and overuse; or the condition may be idiopathic [3–7]. It can lead to severe pain when climbing stairs, ambulating, or even bending the knee [5,8].

Various methods have been attempted for treatment of isolated patellofemoral arthritis. Nonoperative therapy, including strengthening exercises, braces, and nonsteroidal anti-inflammatory medications, may alleviate symptoms, although these treatments have not been shown to slow or stop the progression of arthritis [5,8]. Surgical procedures for correction of patellar malalignment, such as lateral retinacular release, anterior advancement of the tibial tuberosity, and anteromedialization of the tibial tubercle, are treatment options but may not alleviate symptoms or improve quality of life in patients who have advanced arthritis [5,9,10]. Cartilage stimulation procedures such as microfracture and abrasion arthroplasty cause the growth of fibrocartilage on the articular surface, but fibrocartilage in this location is inferior to hyaline cartilage [5,8,11]. Cartilage replacement techniques such as mosaicplasties, autologous chondrocyte implantations, and osteochondral allograft transplant surgeries have been performed but have variable results, with a relatively high failure rate in the patellofemoral joint, and have not been examined in older patients [11–15]. Patellectomy formerly was performed for advanced patellofemoral arthritis, but it has fallen out of favor because of the resultant difficulty with knee flexion and extension [4,9,11]. Patellar resurfacing also has shown poor results [3,4,16,17].

Total knee arthroplasty (TKA) has been a relatively successful treatment for patients who typically are over 60 years of age and for whom other therapies for patellofemoral arthritis have been unsuccessful [9,18–21]. Other authors have advocated patellofemoral arthroplasty (PFA) because it spares healthy bone as well as soft tissues and can easily be revised to a TKA in the case of failure [3–6,22–27].

This article discusses when a TKA should be performed instead of a PFA and, conversely, when a PFA should be performed instead of a TKA. Most of this discussion focuses on patients who are over 60 years of age, because TKAs often are avoided in younger patients. The authors analyzed the results of TKAs and PFAs for isolated patellofemoral arthritis as described in the literature to try to determine the indications and contraindications for these procedures.

* Corresponding author.
 E-mail addresses: rhondamont@aol.com, mmont@lifebridgehealth.org (M.A. Mont).

Literature review

A literature search was performed using the Medline database to find recent studies of PFAs and TKAs performed for isolated patellofemoral arthritis. Peer-reviewed articles were selected for this report if they evaluated at least 15 patients, had a follow-up duration of at least 1 year, and reported the preoperative diagnosis, the revision rate, as well as the reasons for revision.

Eight recent studies were found that evaluated the results of PFA with follow-up times ranging from 1.7 to 20 years [3,4,6,7,23,26–28]. Five reports analyzing the results of TKAs for isolated patellofemoral arthritis, with follow-up times ranging from 2 to 7 years, were assessed [9,18–21]. Tables 1 and 2 show the details of the PFA and the TKA studies, respectively.

Indications and contraindications for patellofemoral arthroplasty

The most common indication for PFA given in the literature was advanced primary isolated patellofemoral arthritis or chondromalacia that severely affected activities of daily living and was not relieved by conservative measures (67% of knees) [3,4,6,7,23,26–28]. Fig. 1 shows an example of advanced primary isolated patellofemoral arthritis. Other indications included patellofemoral arthritis secondary to trochlear dysplasia, chronic subluxation, or recurrent dislocations. Posttraumatic patellofemoral arthritis, most often resulting from patellar fracture, was another indication for PFA. Nonoperative treatments such as physical therapy and analgesics had been unsuccessful in all the patients. In many of these cases, procedures such as lateral retinacular release, anterior tibial tubercle plasty, or patellectomy had been performed but had not produced satisfactory results. Box 1 lists all indications described in the reviewed articles.

PFA was contraindicated, and TKA was performed, if arthritic disease was present in either compartment of the tibiofemoral joint, as illustrated in Figs. 2 and 3. Patella infera also was a contraindication to PFA. Sisto and Sarin [27] excluded patients who were older than 55 years of age, but the other studies did not consider age to be a contraindication. Box 1 lists all the other contraindications listed in the studies and includes conditions that would preclude any joint replacement.

The indication listed in all of the TKA studies was severe isolated patellofemoral arthritis that hindered activities of daily living and was refractory to at least 6 months of conservative treatment [9,18–21]. No other indications were given explicitly, although studies focused on older patients. Contraindications for the TKAs included infection and neuropathic conditions. The presence of radiographically identifiable tibiofemoral arthritis excluded patients from the study groups because the goal was to evaluate isolated patellofemoral arthritis. Indications and contraindications for TKA as described in the literature are listed in Box 2.

Outcomes of patellofemoral arthroplasty for isolated patellofemoral arthritis

As shown in Table 1, the survival rate of PFAs ranged from 95% to 100% at a mean follow-up time of 5 years and then dropped steadily to 85% to 90% at 7 to 8 years, 75% at 10 years, and 58% at 16 years [3,4,6,7,23,26–28]. More than 99% of the failures were attributed to progression of osteoarthritis in the tibiofemoral compartments, and these knees were revised to TKAs. In addition to the revisions, 6% to 44% of the patients experienced joint pain and had arthritic changes in the tibiofemoral compartments 5 to 7 years following the PFAs.

Survival of the PFA was associated strongly with three preoperative characteristics: the presence of trochlear dysplasia, a neutral or nearly neutral Q angle, and a prior patella fracture [3,4,7]. Argenson and colleagues [3] found that 8 of 18 patients who had primary patellofemoral arthritis experienced progression of the disease in the tibiofemoral joint, but only 3 of 21 patients who had preoperative patellar dislocations and 3 of 18 patients who had posttraumatic patellofemoral arthritis developed tibiofemoral arthritis. Nicol and colleagues [7] found that none of the 11 patients who had preoperative trochlear dysplasia required revisions at 7 years, but 5 of 31 patients who did not have trochlear dysplasia required revisions for tibiofemoral osteoarthritis. Cartier and colleagues [4] found that only 6 of 40 patients who had a hip-knee-ankle axis between 177° and 183° experienced progression of tibiofemoral arthritis. All 19 patients who had a hip-knee-ankle axis less than 177° or greater than 183° had developed tibiofemoral arthritis at final follow-up, however [4]. Fig. 4 shows a patient had an abnormal mechanical axis. Patients who had preoperative trochlear dysplasia or who had posttraumatic arthritis associated with a previous

Table 1
Outcomes of patellofemoral arthroplasty for isolated patellofemoral arthritis

Authors	Number of knees/ patients	Mean age in years (range)	Follow-up duration in years (range)	Results
Ackroyd & Chir [22]	109/85	68 (46–86)	5.2 (5–8)	26 knees lost to follow-up. 5.8% survival rate at 5 years for knees that were followed. Median Bristol pain score: 35 of 40 points. Median Oxford knee score: 39 of 48 points. 11 knees revised between 5 and 8 years.
Leadbetter et al [28]	30/25	48 (25–73)	3.25 (0.3–10)	93% survival rate. 25 knees were rated as good to excellent. No validated knee scores were given.
Sisto and Sarin [27]	25/22	45 (23–51)	6.1 (2.7–9.9)	100% survival rate. 18 excellent and 7 good results. The mean Knee Society objective and functional scores were 91 and 89 points, respectively, at final follow-up.
Nicol et al [7]	103/79	68 (46–84)	7.1 (5.5–8.5)	86% survival rate. 7% of surviving arthroplasties had medial compartment osteoarthritis progression.
Argenson et al [3]	66/66	57 (21–82)	16.2 (12–20)	58% survival rate. Mean Knee Society objective and functional scores were 78.5 and 81.2 points, respectively, at final follow-up. Patients who underwent PFA for instability had best results, and patients who had primary arthritis had highest revision rate.
Cartier et al [4]	79/70	60 (36–81)	10 (6–16)	75% survival rate. At final follow-up, Knee Society functional scores were 72% excellent, 19% fair, and 9% failures. Knee Society objective scores were 77% excellent, 14% fair, and 9 failures.
Merchant [26]	16/16	47 (26–81)	4.5 (2.75–6.25)	100% survival rate. 94% of patients reported ADL scores > 70 points at final follow-up.
Merchant [6]	15/15	48.8 (30–81)	3.75 (2.25–5.5)	100% survival rate. 93% of patients reported ADL scores > 70 points at final follow-up. Mean ADL score was 81 points.

Abbreviations: ADL, activities of daily living; PFA, patellofemoral arthroplasty.

patellar fracture were unlikely to experience progressive tibiofemoral arthritis [3,4,7].

Other complications were reported for PFAs. Up to 20% of patients underwent revisions for loosening of the components in one study [3], but the other studies reported no radiographic signs of loosening at 5 to 7 years [4,6,7,23,26–28]. Three percent to 10% of patients required secondary lateral releases for lateral patellar pain following the arthroplasty and subsequently did well [3,4]. One percent to 10% of patients underwent successful manipulations for knee stiffness [3,23].

Outcomes of total knee arthroplasty for isolated patellofemoral arthritis

Overall results for TKA for isolated patellofemoral arthritis were excellent at short- to mid-term

Table 2
Outcomes of total knee arthroplasty for isolated patellofemoral arthritis

Authors	Number of knees/ patients	Mean age in years (range)	Follow-up duration in years (range)	Results
Dalury [18]	33/25	70.2 (54–81)	5.2 (3.8–8.4)	100% survival. Mean Knee Society pain and function scores were 48 and 96 points, respectively.
Mont et al [9]	30/27	73 (59–88)	6.75 (4–11)	100% survival. Mean Knee Society objective and functional scores were 93 and 86 points, respectively. Two patients had occasional anterior knee pain.
Parvizi et al [20]	31/24	70 (47–85)	5.2 (2–12)	94% survival. Mean Knee Society objective and functional scores were 88.9 and 89.5 points, respectively. Five patients had mild anterior knee pain, and one patient had moderate pain.
Thompson et al [21]	33/31	73 (58–89)	1.7 (1–3.3)	100% survival. At final follow-up, 21 knees were pain free, and 12 had occasional anterior pain. No objective score was used.
Laskin & van Steijn [19]	53/53	67 (54–85)	7.4 (3–9.5)	Three patients lost to follow-up, 1 above-knee amputation, 1 revision. 98% survival. Mean Knee Society pain and functional scores were 47 and 96 points, respectively. Three patients had anterior knee pain.

follow-up. Laskin and van Steijn [19] reported 98% survival, with mean Knee Society pain and function scores of 47 and 96 points, respectively, at a mean follow-up of 7.4 years. Thompson and colleagues [21] reported 100% survival with minimal or no pain in 33 knees at a mean follow-up of 1.7 years. Parvizi and colleagues [20] reported 94% survival with mean Knee Society objective and function scores of 88.9 and 89.5 points, respectively, at a follow-up time of

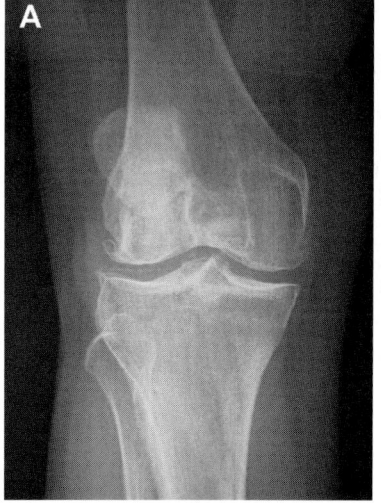 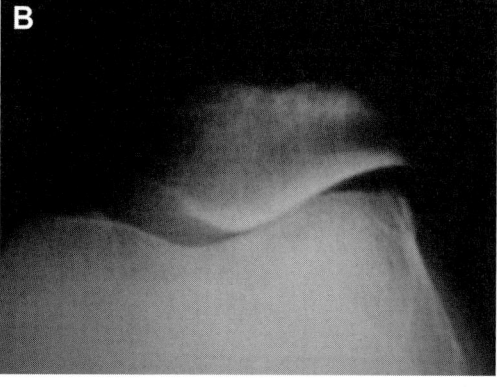

Fig. 1. A 36-year-old patient has (A) a normal tibiofemoral joint and (B) a subluxed patella with patellofemoral arthritis. This patient is a candidate for a patellofemoral arthroplasty.

> **Box 1. Indications and contraindications for patellofemoral arthroplasty**
>
> *Indications*
> Advanced isolated primary patellofemoral arthritis
> Patellofemoral arthritis with trochlear dysplasia
> Early patellofemoral arthritis with failure of alignment procedure
> Posttraumatic isolated patellofemoral arthritis
> Recurrent patellofemoral joint dislocation or subluxation
> Failure of nonoperative treatment
>
> *Contraindications*
> Presence of arthritis at tibiofemoral joint
> Patella infera
> Inflammatory arthritis
> Complex regional pain syndrome
> Infection
> Debilitated patient

5.2 years. Mont and colleagues [9] reported 100% survival with mean Knee Society objective and function scores of 93 and 86 points, respectively, at a mean follow-up time of 6.75 years. Dalury [18] reported 100% survival, with mean Knee Society pain and function scores of 48 and 96 points, respectively, at a mean follow-up time of 5.2 years. Table 2 lists the outcomes of these reports.

Few complications were reported for TKAs performed for isolated patellofemoral arthritis in patients who had a mean age of 67 to 73 years [9,18–21]. Thompson and colleagues [21] reported that 36% of the patients had occasional anterior knee discomfort at a mean follow-up time of 20 months. Parvizi and colleagues [20] reported that 17% of patients had mild and 3% had moderate anterior knee pain at a mean follow-up time of 5 years. Laskin and van Steijn [19] and Mont and colleagues [9] both reported that 6% to 7% of patients experienced mild anterior knee pain at a follow-up time of approximately 7 years. In all the studies, components were well fixed, and no revisions had been performed at up to 12 years following the procedures.

Comparison of patellofemoral arthroplasty and total knee arthroplasty studies

All of the studies examined knees that had severe arthritis of the patellofemoral joint with minimal or no tibiofemoral arthritis. The patients who were treated with TKAs were generally older (mean age, 70.1 years) than the patients who were treated by PFA (mean age, 60.2 years). The mean follow-up duration was 8.3 years for the PFA studies and 5.5 years for the TKA studies. Three of the PFA studies stratified the outcomes by various preoperative diagnoses [3,4,7]. None of the studies stratified the results by age, gender,

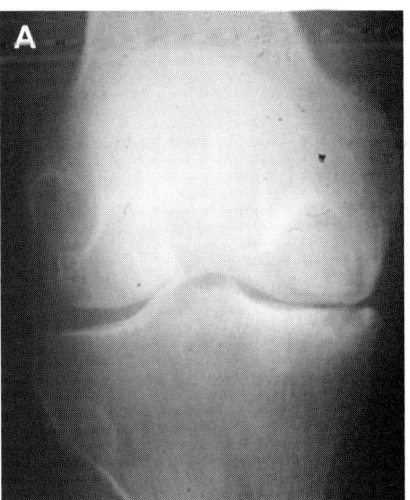 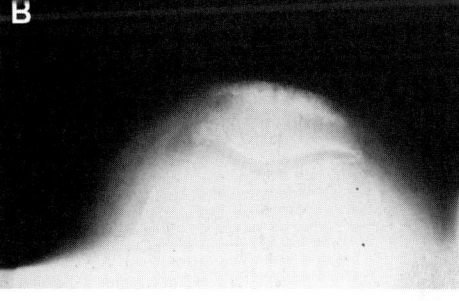

Fig. 2. A 59-year-old patient has osteoarthritis of the (*A*) tibiofemoral and (*B*) patellofemoral joints. This patient is not a candidate for a patellofemoral arthroplasty because of his tricompartmental arthritis and advanced age.

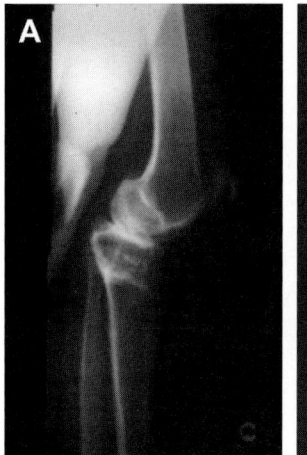
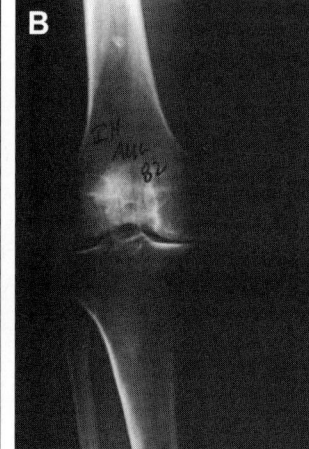

Fig. 3. A 55-year-old patient has (*A*) pseudosubluxation and (*B*) osteoarthritis of the tibiofemoral joint in addition to patellofemoral arthritis. This patient is not a candidate for a patellofemoral arthroplasty because of his tibiofemoral arthritis and instability as well as his age.

body mass index, activity level, or by any other grouping.

Comparison of the functional results of the two procedures reveals few differences. The mean flexion ranges of motion at final follow-up across all of the reports were 116° and 115.6° for PFA and TKA, respectively. Many of the knee scores were not comparable because of varying scoring systems and follow-up times. Sisto and Sarin [27] reported mean Knee Society functional and objective scores of 89 and 91 points, respectively, for the PFAs at a mean follow-up time of 6.1 years. Argenson [3] reported mean Knee Society functional and objective scores of 81.2 and 78.5 points, respectively, for PFAs at a mean follow-up time of 16 years. The TKA studies reported Knee Society pain scores ranging from 47 to 48 points, objective scores ranging from 88.9 to 93 points, and function scores ranging from 89.5 to 96 points at 5.2 to 7.4 years. Table 2 lists these results.

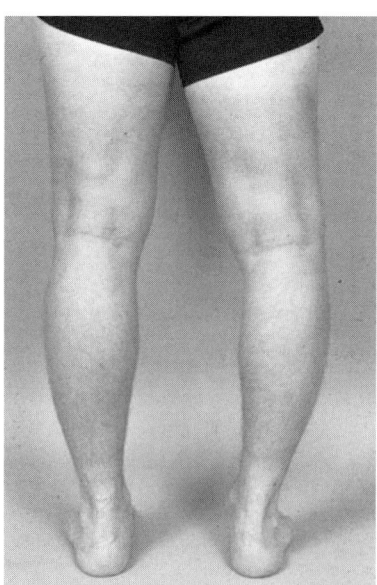

Fig. 4. A 42-year-old patient has an abnormal mechanical axis in addition to patellofemoral arthritis. This patient is not a candidate for a patellofemoral arthroplasty, because patellofemoral arthroplasty is associated with inferior results compared with a total knee arthroplasty in patients who have an abnormal mechanical axis.

Box 2. Indications and contraindications for total knee arthroplasty

Indications
Advanced primary patellofemoral arthritis
Age greater than 60 years
Presence of arthritis in tibiofemoral compartments

Contraindications
Infection
Complex regional pain syndrome
Other causes of knee pain
Debilitated patient

Discussion

PFAs have been performed since the late 1970s. Early designs had a relatively high failure rate [28]. Newer designs have improved alignment, reduced loosening, and decreased patellar maltracking [5,27,28]. At present, the most common reason for failure of PFA is progression of osteoarthritis in the tibiofemoral joint. One way to reduce failure from this cause and to improve patient outcome is to identify the knees that are most likely to benefit or to fail as a result of this procedure and to treat these knees appropriately. The authors conducted this study to determine the parameters that affect the success or failure of PFAs and TKAs performed to treat patellofemoral arthritis.

On the basis of this analysis of the results of PFAs and TKAs in the literature, the authors believe that the indications for PFA include isolated patellofemoral arthritis secondary to congenital trochlear dysplasia or patellar fracture. The knees of patients who were diagnosed with these conditions were least likely to progress to multicompartmental arthritis. PFA is indicated in cases of severe arthritis that inhibits activities of daily living when nonoperative treatment methods have failed. Recurrent patellar dislocations are another indication for this procedure. Additionally, PFA had greater success in patients younger than 60 years, because PFA is a bone-conserving option that can be revised to a TKA if the arthritis does progress to other compartments [5,10,25,27].

As a corollary, one should not perform a PFA for a patient who has any arthritic disease in the tibiofemoral compartments at presentation. Other contraindications for PFA include patella infera and abnormal mechanical axes ($> 3°$ in either direction), because these conditions have been associated with poor outcomes. Both conditions can be corrected surgically before performing PFA, but the authors know of no data regarding the success of PFA following such correction. Additionally, inflammatory arthritis is a contraindication for PFA because of the likelihood of subsequent pain from the tibiofemoral joint.

The indications for TKA as a treatment for severe patellofemoral arthritis include radiographic evidence of tibiofemoral arthritis or inflammatory arthritis and, in patients older than 60 years, severe patellofemoral arthritis. The age demarcation between the choice of a PFA versus a TKA has not been resolved. With further data including larger studies of PFAs with longer follow-up times, indications may be expanded further.

Summary

Patients who have patellofemoral arthritis secondary to trochlear dysplasia or a prior patellar fracture often continue to do well at 5 to 15 years following PFA. Patients who have malalignment at the knee joint, manifested by patella infera or an increased Q angle, do worse after PFA than other patients, although the results after surgical correction are not known. Patients who are at a higher risk for development of arthritis in other compartments (eg, those who have inflammatory arthritis) frequently require a revision to a TKA after 5 to 7 years. Patients who are over 60 years of age have a higher likelihood of developing tibiofemoral arthritis sooner and are less likely to need a temporizing procedure. Because the range of motion achieved with TKAs is similar to that achieved with PFAs, and because TKAs have a higher function score and a lower failure rate than PFAs, the authors believe that they now are a better option for older patients. Future studies that stratify patients by age, gender, anatomic variation, and preoperative diagnosis may elucidate further appropriate indications and contraindications for these procedures.

References

[1] McAlindon TE, Snow S, Cooper C, et al. Radiographic patterns of osteoarthritis of the knee joint in the community: the importance of the patellofemoral joint. Ann Rheum Dis 1992;51(7):844–9.

[2] Davies AP, Vince AS, Shepstone L, et al. The radiologic prevalence of patellofemoral osteoarthritis. Clin Orthop Relat Res 2002;402:206–12.

[3] Argenson JN, Flecher X, Parratte S, et al. Patellofemoral arthroplasty: an update. Clin Orthop Relat Res 2005;440:50–3.

[4] Cartier P, Sanouiller JL, Khefacha A. Long-term results with the first patellofemoral prosthesis. Clin Orthop Relat Res 2005;436:47–54.

[5] Lonner JH. Patellofemoral arthroplasty. J Am Acad Orthop Surg 2007;15(8):495–506.

[6] Merchant AC. Early results with a total patellofemoral joint replacement arthroplasty prosthesis. J Arthroplasty 2004;19(7):829–36.

[7] Nicol SG, Loveridge JM, Weale AE, et al. Arthritis progression after patellofemoral joint replacement. Knee 2006;13(4):290–5.

[8] Lotke PA, Lonner JH, Nelson CL. Patellofemoral arthroplasty: the third compartment. J Arthroplasty 2005;20(4 Suppl 2):4–6.

[9] Mont MA, Haas S, Mullick T, et al. Total knee arthroplasty for patellofemoral arthritis. J Bone Joint Surg Am 2002;84-A(11):1977–81.

[10] Newman JH. Patellofemoral arthritis and its management with isolated patellofemoral replacement: a personal experience. Orthopedics 2007;30(Suppl 8):58–61.

[11] Fulkerson JP. Alternatives to patellofemoral arthroplasty. Clin Orthop Relat Res 2005;436:76–80.

[12] Hangody L, Fules P. Autologous osteochondral mosaicplasty for the treatment of full-thickness defects of weight-bearing joints: ten years of experimental and clinical experience. J Bone Joint Surg Am 2003;85-A(Suppl 2):25–32.

[13] Torga Spak R, Teitge RA. Fresh osteochondral allografts for patellofemoral arthritis: long-term followup. Clin Orthop Relat Res 2006;444:193–200.

[14] Jamali AA, Emmerson BC, Chung C, et al. Fresh osteochondral allografts. Clin Orthop Relat Res 2005;437:176–85.

[15] Minas T, Bryant T. The role of autologous chondrocyte implantation in the patellofemoral joint. Clin Orthop Relat Res 2005;436:30–9.

[16] Insall J, Tria AJ, Aglietti P. Resurfacing of the patella. J Bone Joint Surg Am 1980;62(6):933–6.

[17] Worrell RV. Resurfacing of the patella in young patients. Orthop Clin North Am 1986;17(2):303–9.

[18] Dalury DF. Total knee replacement for patellofemoral disease. J Knee Surg 2005a;18(4):274–7.

[19] Laskin RS, van Steijn M. Total knee replacement for patients with patellofemoral arthritis. Clin Orthop Relat Res 1999;367:89–95.

[20] Parvizi J, Stuart MJ, Pagnano MW, et al. Total knee arthroplasty in patients with isolated patellofemoral arthritis. Clin Orthop Relat Res 2001;392:147–52.

[21] Thompson NW, Ruiz AL, Breslin E, et al. Total knee arthroplasty without patellar resurfacing in isolated patellofemoral osteoarthritis. J Arthroplasty 2001;16(5):607–12.

[22] Ackroyd CE, Chir B. Development and early results of a new patellofemoral arthroplasty. Clin Orthop Relat Res 2005;436:7–13.

[23] Ackroyd CE, Newman JH, Evans R, et al. The Avon patellofemoral arthroplasty: five-year survivorship and functional results. J Bone Joint Surg Br 2007;89(3):310–5.

[24] Clyburn TA, Weitz-Marshall A, Ambrose CM, et al. Outcomes of patellofemoral replacement in total knee arthroplasty using meticulous techniques. Orthopedics 2007;30(2):111–5.

[25] Lonner JH, Jasko JG, Booth RE Jr. Revision of a failed patellofemoral arthroplasty to a total knee arthroplasty. J Bone Joint Surg Am 2006;88(11):2337–42.

[26] Merchant AC. A modular prosthesis for patellofemoral arthroplasty: design and initial results. Clin Orthop Relat Res 2005;436:40–6.

[27] Sisto DJ, Sarin VK. Custom patellofemoral arthroplasty of the knee. J Bone Joint Surg Am 2006;88(7):1475–80.

[28] Leadbetter WB, Seyler TM, Ragland PS, et al. Indications, contraindications, and pitfalls of patellofemoral arthroplasty. J Bone Joint Surg Am 2006;88(Suppl 4):122–37.

Index

Note: Page numbers of article titles are in **boldface** type.

A

ACI. See *Autologous chondrocyte implantation (ACI).*

AMZ. See *Anteromedialization (AMZ).*

Anterior knee pain, diagnoses related to, factors cited in literature for association with, 288–289

Anteromedialization (AMZ)
 ACI with, in patellofemoral chondrosis management, **329–335**. See also *Patellofemoral chondrosis, management of, AMZ with ACI in.*
 described, 329–331

Arthritis. See also *Patellofemoral arthritis.*
 inflammatory, osteoarthritis and, 273
 patellofemoral. See *Patellofemoral arthritis.*

Arthroplasty, patellofemoral. See *Patellofemoral arthroplasty.*

Articular cartilage
 evaluation of, in patellofemoral syndrome, 301
 of patella, 269

Autologous chondrocyte implantation (ACI), AMZ with, in patellofemoral chondrosis management, **329–335**. See also *Patellofemoral chondrosis, management of, AMZ with ACI in.*

Avon patellofemoral arthroplasty (PFA) prosthesis, 364

C

Cartilage
 articular
  evaluation of, in patellofemoral syndrome, 301
  of patella, 269
 failure mode of, 293

D

Degenerative pain, patellofemoral, operative treatment of, limitations of, 364–367

Dislocation(s), patellar, recurrent, management of, **313–327**. See also *Patellar dislocation, recurrent, management of.*

Dysplasia, patellofemoral, patellofemoral arthritis due to, 270–272

E

Exercise(s)
 mobilization, 277
 resistive, pain-free, progression quadriceps strengthening for, 277
 stretching, 277

F

Focal anatomic patellofemoral inlay resurfacing, **337–346**. See also *Patellofemoral inlay resurfacing, focal anatomic.*

G

Genetic(s), patellofemoral arthritis and, 273

I

Inflammatory arthritis, osteoarthritis and, 273

Instability, patellar
 biomechanics of, 314
 pathoanatomies of, 318

K

Knee pain, anterior, diagnoses related to, factors cited in literature for association with, 288–289

L

Ligament(s)
 failure mode of, 293
 patellofemoral, evaluation of, in patellofemoral syndrome, 300–301

M

Malalignment, patellofemoral arthritis due to, 269–270

Mobilization exercises, 277

Muscle(s)
 failure mode of, 293
 in patellofemoral syndrome, evaluation of, 301

Muscle strength considerations, before advocating operative care, 278–282

O

Obesity, patellofemoral arthritis due to, 272–273

Osteoarthritis, inflammatory arthritis and, 273

P

Pain
- degenerative, patellofemoral, operative treatment of, limitations of, 364–367
- knee, anterior, diagnoses related to, factors cited in literature for association with
- levels of
  - categories of, 275
  - in patellofemoral rehabilitation, 275–277

Patella
- articular cartilage of, 269
- malalignment of, 269–270

Patella alta, 321

Patellar dislocation
- epidemiology of, 313–314
- incidence of, 313
- natural history of, 313–314
- recurrent
  - described, 313
  - management of, **313–327**
    - historic, 317
    - minimally invasive patellar realignment in, 322–323
    - MPFL reconstruction in, 319–321
    - nonsurgical, 317–318
    - pathoanatomy approach in, 318–322
    - postoperative, 323
    - proximal patellar realignment in, 319
    - soft-tissue realignment in, 319
    - surgical, 317–322
  - patient history in, 314–315
  - physical examination in, 315–316
  - radiographic findings in, 316–317

Patellar instability
- biomechanics of, 314
- pathoanatomies of, 318

Patellar tracking
- in patellofemoral syndrome, 292–293
- patellofemoral arthroplasty design features affecting, 347–349

Patellofemoral arthritis
- dysplasia and, 270–272
  - instability and, 272
- genetic components of, 273
- isolated
  - knee pain and, 381
  - TKA for
    - outcomes of, 383–385
    - results of, **381–388**. See also *Total knee arthroplasty (TKA), for isolated patellofemoral arthritis.*
- malalignment and, 269–270
- obesity and, 272–273
- patellofemoral arthroplasty for, **363–379**. See also *Patellofemoral arthroplasty, for patellofemoral arthritis.*
- pathophysiology of, **269–274**
- trauma and, 272

Patellofemoral arthroplasty
- contraindications to, **381–388**
- design of, outcomes related to, **347–354**
  - clinical results–related, 349–352
  - complications, 349–352
  - patellar tracking–related, 347–349
  - Zimmer Gender Solutions PFJ, 352–353
- for isolated patellofemoral arthritis, outcomes of, 382–383
- for patellofemoral arthritis, **363–379**
  - contraindications to, 367–370
  - recommendations related to, 370–376
- indications for, 382
- novel applications of, 376–377
- TKA vs., studies of, 385–386
- with customized trochlear prosthesis, **355–362**
  - clinical experience with, 358
  - contraindications to, 356
  - design rationale for, 355–356
  - indications for, 356
  - keys to success with, 360–361
  - surgical technique, 358–360

Patellofemoral chondrosis, management of, AMZ with ACI in, **329–335**
- discussion of, 333–335
- operative technique, 331–332
- results of, 333–335

Patellofemoral degenerative pain, operative treatment of, limitations of, 364–367

Patellofemoral disease
- causes of, 275, 276
- prevalence of, 355
- treatment of, factors guiding, 337

Patellofemoral dysplasia, patellofemoral arthritis due to, 270–272

Patellofemoral inlay resurfacing, focal anatomic, **337–346**
case reports, 340–343
contraindications to, 338
described, 337–338
discussion of, 343–344
indications for, 338
patient assessment in, 338
surgical technique, 338–340

Patellofemoral ligament, evaluation of, in patellofemoral syndrome, 300–301

Patellofemoral rehabilitation
before advocating operative care, **275–285**
muscle strength considerations, 278–282
soft tissue flexibility considerations, 277–278
taping and, 282–284
pain level in determination of, 275–277

Patellofemoral syndrome, **287–311**
anatomy related to, 294–295
biomechanics of, 293–294
case study analysis in, 305–310
described, 287
evaluation of
articular cartilage in, 301
muscles in, 301
patellofemoral ligament in, 300–301
skeleton in, 295–300
tendons in, 301
literature review of, 287–290
patellar tracking in, 292–293
scientific knowledge about, 290–292
surgical treatments for, 303–304

PFA prosthesis. See *Avon patellofemoral arthroplasty (PFA) prosthesis.*

Progression quadriceps strengthening, for pain-free resistive exercise, 277

Prosthesis(es)
Avon PKA, 364
trochlear, customized, patellofemoral arthroplasty with, **355–362**. See also *Patellofemoral arthroplasty, with customized trochlear prosthesis.*

Q

Quadriceps, strengthening of, pain-free resistive exercise for, 277

R

Radiography, in recurrent patellar dislocation, 316–317

Recurrent patellar dislocation, management of, **313–327**. See also *Patellar dislocation, recurrent, management of.*

Rehabilitation, patellofemoral, before advocating operative care, 275–285. See also *Patellofemoral rehabilitation, before advocating operative care.*

Resistive exercise, pain-free, progression quadriceps strengthening for, 277

S

Skeleton
evaluation of, in patellofemoral syndrome, 295–300
failure mode of, 293

Soft tissue flexibility considerations, before advocating operative care, 277–278

Stretching exercise, 277

T

Taping, patellar, 282–284

Tendon(s)
failure mode of, 293
in patellofemoral syndrome, evaluation of, 301

TKA. See *Total knee arthroplasty (TKA).*

Total knee arthroplasty (TKA)
for isolated patellofemoral arthritis
discussion of, 387
indications for, 382
literature review related to, 382
outcomes of, 382–383
results of, **381–388**
patellofemoral arthroplasty vs., studies of, 385–386

Total knee replacement. See *Total knee arthroplasty (TKA).*

Trauma, patellofemoral arthritis due to, 272

Trochlear prosthesis, customized, patellofemoral arthroplasty with, **355–362**. See also *Patellofemoral arthroplasty, with customized trochlear prosthesis.*

Z

Zimmer Gender Solutions PFJ, design features of, 352–353

Moving?

Make sure your subscription moves with you!

To notify us of your new address, find your **Clinics Account Number** (located on your mailing label above your name), and contact customer service at:

E-mail: elspcs@elsevier.com

800-654-2452 (subscribers in the U.S. & Canada)
1-407-563-6020 (subscribers outside of the U.S. & Canada)

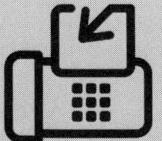

Fax number: 407-363-9661

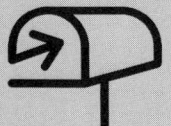

Elsevier Periodicals Customer Service
6277 Sea Harbor Drive
Orlando, FL 32887-4800

*To ensure uninterrupted delivery of your subscription, please notify us at least 4 weeks in advance of move.

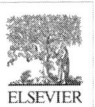